Inching Back To Sane, 2nd Edition

Copyright Leif Gregersen, February 2017

www.edmontonwriter.com

viking3082000@yahoo.com

written by: Leif Gregersen

edited by: Richard Van Camp, Alanna Campbell

This book is dedicated first to my Dad, who never stopped caring, second to Richard Van Camp who never stopped encouraging, and to Charity Slobod who never stopped inspiring. Without these three people this book would never have gone to print.

All the best!

Remember, there is always hope!

Other Works by Leif Gregersen

Poetry:

-Poems From Inside Me

-First White of Winter Poems

-Stargazer: My Life in Constellations

-Poetry of Love, Life and Hope

Short Stories:

-The Base Jumpers and Other Stories

-Mustang Summer

Young Adult Novels:

-In the Blink of an Eye, a Journey Through Time

-Those Who Dare To Dream

Table of Contents:

4

Chapter one: Old Problems, New Beginnings

Back in 1991 to 1992 I lived in Vancouver at the age of 19 and 20 years old. There I experienced fun and carefree times like never before, but it wasn't ever destined to be paradise. The building I lived in for most of that time was a youth hostel that was more of a rooming house for young travelers, and I had so many interesting and cool friends. Matt was one guy I got along well with. He was the hostel manager. He had a kick-ass stereo system, and he was always blasting only the best music. There was this song that had come out only a few months before that he played a lot; it totally blew me away, it was Tom Cochrane's "Life is a Highway," and it always got me going. It talked about Vancouver right along with far-flung, exotic places. Every time I heard it, it reminded me of the long runs I used to take around Stanley Park and how I could see five or six different viewpoints of the Vancouver skyline, from the north shore to downtown to the west end and a few more viewpoints in total darkness out to sea.

Every night was a party in that hostel, beer was cheap back then, and there was always someone generous enough to buy. Sometimes we would play poker for quarters and dimes, and sometimes we would just get sit around and swap stories. A lot of Australians couldn't believe things about northern Canada, and a lot of Canadians couldn't conceive of some things about Australians like how they treated their women, and consumed their beer.

That summer was probably the best of my life. I had found freedom; I had found a career path I was excited about. Most of the time I was taking flying lessons I paid for through a student loan to get my professional license a couple of days a week. Flying those planes and feeling I had a great future in store for me gave me a lot of confidence. I was meeting so many women, likely because of feeling so good about myself. My nights were often spent laying in the top bunk of my bed with the cool summer harbor front breeze coming in through the open window. I had no worries then. I had nothing to steal worth anything, and most of the thieves would focus on breaking into cars further up Grouse Mountain or in West Vancouver. I entered and left my room through the open window whenever I felt like going anywhere, and never bothered to closing or locking it.

There was an amazing radio station called "The Fox, " that played all the hits. I would leave it playing all night while I dreamed along with the tunes. Songs like "Take on Me" by Aha, "The Boxer" by Paul Simon, or "For the Longest Time" by Billy Joel would drift into my subconscious while I was asleep. I would bask in the celebration and beauty that pop music was back then. Popular music just seemed to have so much more meaning in the early 90s. It either talked about love or travel or the things the world had in store for the young people that listened to it. Sometimes it would take a stand against war or injustice. I can't listen to a lot of the new stuff these days, it just doesn't seem to have the same soul.

Most of the time when it came to music, I was a 100% Bruce Springsteen fan. As I walked through the metropolis of Vancouver, I would play all the songs of his I loved over in my mind. When I had a car with a good sound system in it back home, I would sing out loud while I was driving. Everything back then was set to the tune of a song by him it seemed. I felt a real connection to Bruce, and later I found out that he suffered from depression which comes out in a lot of his work and is also something which was prevalent in my family. I had a couple of his tapes when I lived on the coast. The one that meant the most to me was "Tunnel of Love, " but I was also into his older, brooding stuff like the "Nebraska" album where he sang songs about guys going on rampages and killing themselves. My brother used to say that "Born in the USA" was the one album he made for his fans, but to me all Springsteen is good Springsteen. The Nebraska album was the kind of artistry that was both dark and beautiful, and I ate it up. At different points in my life, I owned every album he had put out. Sometimes I would lay back in the dark and play his music loud on the headphones, and it was almost like I could channel Bruce through the music. I always felt like his biggest fan, even though millions loved him.

As my stay on the coast was ending, I went to see the movie "Terminator 2, " and it seemed to unbalance my mind. It wasn't the first movie with Arnold in it to do so either, a while back I was in a mental institution in Alberta, and they played "Total Recall" for the patients, and I was in such a sad state of mind I thought the fictional special effects in it were real. "Terminator 2" was even worse because the main character in that show was in a mental hospital and had to escape to keep the evil Terminator from killing her son with the help of a good Terminator that had been re-programmed in the future. As my illness took over, I began thinking that everything around me was a trick played on me in the future, that I had far outlived everyone I knew. I imagined that some big government conspiracy was going on and they had put parts of this movie in a mental hospital to warn me or trap me; I didn't know which. What was scary was that just as some movies were reaching deep down into my psyche, there were some songs that seemed to be telling me secret information. If U2 was on the radio I would begin thinking about being 15 and in love with a girl who would never love me. Only my mind would invent the idea that she was hiding somewhere and had called in to ask that the the song to be played to tell me there still was a chance for a relationship. There were so many songs though and so many women that I had crushes on that everything seemed to mean something. There were even songs that seemed to pull up deep evil impulses from the depths of my being.

As is the nature of psychosis, it seemed with all the false sensory input confusing me, such as playing games, thoughts about aliens coming out of nowhere, that the only logical answer seemed to be they had somehow put my brain into a robot's head and that under my skin was metal. I imagined cameras in my eyes and a computer keeping my ancient heartbeat going. It was lucky I was admitted into a treatment facility before I began trying to claw my skin off.

It's so hard to describe being that sick, the pain, the thoughts, the voices, and the denial. During those times, my digestion was always extremely out of whack. I would have so much disruption in my lower abdomen I sometimes couldn't do anything but sit on the toilet, and try to manage the excruciating pain. Being in active psychosis is like being put through a transporter like in Star Trek except something has gone wrong and your nervous system was delivered a millimeter out of place. The psychosis causes everything to go haywire and all kinds of false information to enter your head from your senses and your brain draws false conclusions and fears appear from nothing. On this night when I felt like I was a robot, with so many conflicting thoughts and ideas coursing through my mind, I decided to walk out to the massive Lion's Gate Bridge connecting West Vancouver with Stanley Park and jump down to the icy waters hundreds of feet below. Somehow part of my mind was working and fought with the crazy half to try and get help. I called the cops, and I was so ashamed of being ill that I told them I thought someone at the hostel had put some hallucinogenic drugs in my food. They took me to a psychiatric ward right then and there.

The hospital in Vancouver treated me well, they have a fantastic system there. The food is top notch, the ward I was on was clean and the staff was flawlessly helpful. They seemed to truly care about what happened to you. I hadn't had an experience like that in the Alberta Hospital in Edmonton. The sad fact of being in this 'nice' hospital was, I think there was a possibility they may have wrongly diagnosed me. Even though I loved Vancouver and wished to stay there, I thought the only option I had left was to go home and go into the hospital with doctors that could help me more. I also had some false ideas that there were relationships and opportunities in Edmonton that would make going back worthwhile. Not to mention it was so hard to go through the experience of being sick without family around me.

Thinking back to the day I packed up all my stuff, gave away what I was unable to carry, and left Vancouver for good, sometimes I think that it would have been better to stay there despite my diminished capacity. Who knows what course my life may have taken? The reality was, though, that I was so ill that I wouldn't have been able to take care of myself in a short amount of time.

I had left the Lion's Gate Hospital in Vancouver with a diagnosis of schizophrenia and enough delusions racing around in my head to believe it was true. As a parting gift from the hospital, they gave me a small amount of medication to counteract the time-release antipsychotic drug, which had been administered by injection. I went back to the hostel where I had lived just before being admitted to Lion's Gate to wait out whatever time I could grab before being sent back to a psychiatric ward again. After I paid a large portion of my monthly disability income to cover the costs of me not living at the hostel, I paid most of what was left of my money for a few more days and hoped that I could somehow make it through.

All the while I was in the hospital in Vancouver, my delusional thoughts and strange ideas were becoming increasingly worse. My actual diagnosis was bipolar disorder with some symptoms of schizophrenia and anxiety. The injectable medication coursing through my veins was simply not working as it should have been.

One day I was alone in my room back at the hostel. For some reason, I believed someone had bugged the room with listening devices, and all kinds of government and spy agencies were listening to me. I started yelling out that I was to be taken aboard a spaceship and given a tattoo signifying I was a pilot. I could hear people laughing at me and making jokes in the next room. One of them came to the door and asked me if I was okay, and I answered, "Oh, I'm just trying to get some records transferred." I wonder if he knew I had lost my mind or perhaps thought I had a cellular phone.

I could often come up with believable lies when people caught me hallucinating. The chance of being caught for being a liar seemed better than being caught as a person with a mental illness. I would say I thought someone had slipped me some drugs or that I was talking into a voice recorder in my pocket. When I think back to that time, I feel incredibly ashamed about the whole thing. Who can trust someone who does and says such things? Thanks to television, the general belief of the public is that people who are mentally ill are out to harm or murder them and that their illnesses are contagious. In my case, my mental illness just filled me with confusion and fear.

I had a roommate who was kind and helpful, and we would often talk about his brother. I was soon hallucinating he was my own brother who had come out to Vancouver to rescue me from these powerful people my paranoid thoughts invented. My psychosis convinced me riches and fame awaited me if I do just some small thing of significance, like walking across the street at a certain time or yelling out a sound. Once while in my room shouting or talking to myself and some guy I didn't know came into my room and unplugged my clock radio, resetting it. He walked out and then made jokes about me with others in the next room and I could hear the laughter through the paper-thin walls of the hostel.

I was to find out years later that a former friend of mine, considered me a psychopath. I had wrongly believed she was going to try and help me through my problems if I returned to Edmonton. Psychopathy was a condition that I was in no way even close to being. A psychopath is completely lacking in a conscience, someone who will murder people, purposely destroying their self-esteem and doing things that most normal people would find horrendous. They will start fires for no reason that causing extreme danger to others (though even for psychopaths this is rare) and not have any bad feelings. What I had was a psychotic delusion. Psychosis is when a person's mind is chemically imbalanced and false ideas, and delusions of grandeur in conjunction with paranoid thoughts occur. In my case, I wouldn't think of harming anyone, much less this young woman who had been a close friend for years.

People who have a mental illness are rarely violent to others but more prone to directing violence at themselves. They are also much more likely to be a victim of violence rather than a perpetrator. Just the other day I was on a bus and saw a disabled older man talking to himself terrified while being picked on by others. He was pushed to the point where he begged the bus driver to call the police. Being mentally ill is frightening to the afflicted person that suffers from it, and 99% of the time they are far from being dangerous.

In Vancouver, a few days passed, and I was feeling the strain of being in a place for young travelers when I likely should have been in an institution. With what I had left of money, I bought a ticket on the bus headed back to Edmonton. One of the reasons I later regretted my decision was that mental health treatment in North Vancouver was so much better than anything in Edmonton. One more example of how much more consumer friendly the system in British Columbia was. When I was in the hospital, they paid a staff member to be a 'buddy' to me. He showed me around, talked to me. He was there to make sure I was taken care of and comfortable. I don't know how a hospital could afford such a thing. To add to that, when I got out, they had a student nurse in a Registered Psychiatric Nursing program call me and check up on me, and she seemed very kind and helpful.

The last thing I did while leaving Vancouver, was ride the sea bus (the harbor ferry connecting the North Shore to Downtown Vancouver). I asked for and got permission to go into the control room and talk to the sea bus drivers. Somehow I managed to hold my words and thoughts together, and I stood beside these men who had the best job in the BC Transit system and helped them with a crossword puzzle as the dazzling skyline of Downtown Vancouver at night grew larger before me. It was breath-taking, and for the first time, I had a perfect front row seat. It pained me to have to leave that beautiful place.

I boarded the cross-Canada bus after buying my ticket for the 1,300-km journey to Edmonton and kept trying to sleep through the ride. It was tough to sit still for all that time. I had some Acetaminophen with me, and I would take a couple of pills and sleep for an hour or two then get up and repeat the process. It was a dangerous game I was playing with my liver, but the problem was that the medication the hospital gave me by injection wouldn't let me rest for a minute. I was also having all kinds of paranoid delusions. There seemed to be no boundaries to my madness: any female was a young woman from my hometown who was disguised and watching me, trying to see if I was following the voices in my head that seemed like orders. Any male who roughly fit the looks of Oliver Stone was spending his millions to get me the help I needed because I had telepathically written an Oscar-winning script for one of his movies. It was obvious that my medication wasn't helping me the way it should have been, but I was tired of running, tired of putting my family through the hell of not knowing what crazy situation they would have to help me out of next. On top of all that, my poor diet and anxiety were working away at my stomach. Having enough food was part of the reason I wanted to go back home to Edmonton. Once, in Vancouver, I was so desperate to eat I did something totally out of character: I stole from a convenience store. It was just a small can of stew, but to me, it was as bad as taking the entire cash register. I was deathly afraid of being caught for that and when I saw pictures in the paper and on TV of thieves on surveillance cameras I was so convinced it was me that I contacted the police thinking they wanted me to turn myself in.

It felt like a long time went by on the bus to Edmonton. It took all night and much of the next day. I believe the trip takes about 18 hours if the bus stops in each small town, which, while cramped into such a small space, seemed like an eternity.

I think it was in Jasper, Alberta, about 350 km from Edmonton, that I called my sister. I tried to convince her and her boyfriend that I needed them to pick me up at the bus station, that I was in a dire situation. I suppose I must have put them through a lot because they didn't want to help me at all at first.

Chapter Two: No Hope and No One To Help

"You have to help me; I think if I don't get some help the worst could happen," I said to my sister's boyfriend in desperation from the payphone at the train station in Jasper. My head at that time was swimming with a cocktail of pills, medicine, and delusional thoughts.

"I will help you but only on one condition!" My sister's boyfriend said.

"Yes, what do you want?"

"I will help you only if you promise me right now that you will never ask me for a single thing again!"

I had no control over being sick, and all I was asking was a ride to a hospital-any hospital, and here he was demanding that I get out of his and my sister's life forever. Just a short while before, my sister was the world to me and all of us were a tight family, spending most of our time together, going to movies, playing sports. I had gone down the drain a long way in such a short time, but there was still hope, there was still a way out if I could admit to my illness and accept treatment. I was ready but unfortunately the mental health treatment system in Edmonton wasn't.

They did come and meet me at the bus station and took me to a hospital. When I got there, I still couldn't sit still for more than a few seconds. Waiting for the doctor to see me, I went out and paced around and smoked, and the two of them walked with me. As this was happening, my psychosis was working away at me, trying to convince me of all kinds of strange things, some of which angered the people with me. All of it was a surreal experience.

They wanted to know why I came there and I mentioned something about a girlfriend and thinking she would help me. By that time, it partially was a hallucination. I had tried to call this person who I thought was a friend two months before. We had some long talks and seemed to connect. My delusions made me believe she was perhaps more than a friend. I got my answer to that question when I tried to call her a few days later, and she wouldn't answer and soon had her number changed to an unlisted one.

After a lot of pacing and waiting, they called me in to wait in a windowless, sterile room to see the doctor, and he came in and talked to me. He said it was a busy time of year and that all the psychiatric beds were full. He didn't seem to understand my desperation and what was going on in my head. One of the staff there said to me that the hospital wasn't a place for a person to get a bed and a shower for the night. I didn't understand what they expected me to do. I could barely sit still and I couldn't even think straight for long enough to properly take care of myself.

That night as far as any treatment or medications went was that a woman came in, took my socks away, threw them in the garbage and then she tried to make a half-assed pair of socks out of thin bandages and tape. These didn't take care of the smell, and they soon fell to pieces, making my feet even colder when I went outside.

As a final suggestion, the hospital staff directed me to a free hostel that I could stay in where I had been before. It was the filthiest, dirtiest roach motel I had ever experienced. It was full of alcoholics, drug addicts, people with sicknesses of every kind, and people who were out of work and desperate. Since then, I have come to view the place in a different way; how they ask no questions and set no standards for helping people. But in all reality, it was the last place a sick person who couldn't take care of themselves would want to go. When I was at a different stage in my recovery from mental illness, I had an occasion to get my hands on a large fruit platter and I went to that same hostel and passed out fresh fruit to everyone in there. It felt good to give something back to a place that had helped me and I have long wanted to do more for them.

The people at the hostel tried to get across that I would be much safer if I could stay with a family member, however I understood my sister's situation. She told him she was a student and that she didn't have the room to keep me at her apartment which was true. My mom and dad had a three-bedroom town house but they had their fill of me. It hurts when I look back at those times and realize that all of them did care and that I had willingly gone off my medication. There were a couple of reasons why I had done this. The first is that many people with my illness experience a symptom known as anosognosia, which means that they are not aware of their own condition. The other thing was that it was so hard to accept all the side effects and limitations that medications place on a person. I suppose there is also the problem that comes when you don't continue to see a psychiatrist on an outpatient basis, you take your medications, start to feel better and then it seems the pills have done their job and are no longer needed. Now, I had to own my illness and I couldn't just rely on my family when I got sick. I didn't say anything to my sister, but I will admit that it hurt. I had done some awful things to her over the years. There was this one time I tried to have her boyfriend deported back to Greece because he assaulted me. There were many times that we would get into screaming arguments as children and I would punch her. I didn't see how I could be in such a situation where no one cared, but as mentioned, it all came down to choices I had made. I am so grateful that my illness didn't take me in other directions making me into a mentally ill and homeless person or a repeat offender in jail for life.

I took my pills as directed, and since I was put down on the sick list they didn't kick me out during the day to look for work. I was allowed to stay inside all day. The food was horrendous in some ways, but I had dropped below 135 pounds since returning from California (in high school I was 170-185, now, over 240) and so I didn't care much about the quality of the food, as long as there was lots of it. I tried to sleep away my days until my sister's friend who had been kind enough to drive me to the hospital without even knowing me when I returned to Edmonton on the bus, came by and visited me and took me out for a coffee a few times.

My sister's friend was one of the most interesting people I knew in Edmonton. His name was Wallace, and he had just one arm. He had no trouble getting around or driving, and he was a very kind and level-headed person. We got to know each other well and one day I shared with him that I had made a pledge to quit drinking on New Year's Eve. He said he went to abstinence groups himself and took me to my first meeting. I was glad to go, but I was still quite delusional, and I often spoke out of turn or said things that didn't make sense, but Wallace kept taking me.

I can't discuss at all what went on in the meetings. It was good for me, I suppose, to get out and talk. But I don't know if there was any real point in me going there other than just talking about myself, at least not back then. As time went on the meetings did help me experience real growth. At the time, though, I was sick, and I wouldn't have drank alcohol even if I had the money for it. The steps that one had to work through in that group where incredible. I will always have a lot of respect for them. They have been adapted into mental health programs and many other types of addictions programs. A man I met in a group once quoted to me from the book they receive their mandates from, he said "We don't have a cure. We have a daily reprieve based on the maintenance of our spiritual condition."

I liked the people I met in meetings. I liked that they had a life philosophy that seemed to work well for many people. I just didn't see how it would work for me, and in my immaturity, I didn't get serious about the meetings for a good number of years. When I did though, I observed immense changes in my life.

While I was in the 'free' hostel, there was a group of about four or five guys who were 'high on God'. They were happy to be there in the shelter; they felt somehow their mission was to come to Edmonton and go on welfare so they could minister to all the heathens. It seemed a bit preposterous. The funny thing, while many people there didn't like their happy attitude in a place that seemed so miserable, I had an urge to be like them. They were all close friends, had each other to rely on and had a glowing aura of innocence to them.

Over the past months that I had lived in Vancouver, I had come to embrace a sort of spirituality, something more akin to a religion of nature like the Native people of Vancouver and other indigenous people. My roommate influenced me a lot. At one time, he had faith in a Judeo-Christian God. He even had a sister who owned a Christian Bookstore who was a helpful and caring person. When I first moved back to Vancouver, she had provided us with some furniture and I would stop at her store now and then and talk about how I dreamed of one day owning a used bookstore.

I had some interesting arguments in the hostel with our local 'God Squad, 'but they didn't change any of my opinions. There was also a man there who would often stand by the door and talk to people from the hostel and invite them to Bible studies and such. Seeing as how we got food that primarily wasn't the healthy and these Bible studies always had snacks, I tried to talk to him to see if I could go to one.

I soon learned the guy was a total ass who thought he had enough life experience to qualify himself as a psychiatrist. If I smoked a small cheap cigar which was just a tobacco leaf wrapped up into the size of a cigarette, somehow word would come to him that I was a drug user. If my eyes were bugged out due to my medications, it added to that and of course since he was so wise in the ways of the world, he had the idea I was also not taking my medications, which was impossible unless I had figured out how to give myself a blood transfusion. There are so many people that care a great deal about the people in shelters and want to help, but this guy only seemed to want to have power over others. It was no surprise that he admitted to spending most of his life in the military.

It was horrible that this man felt he needed to point fingers and make accusations, and do it in the name of religion. One time I even was going to try listening to a sermon at the church he was from, but I got restless and edgy and decided to leave. He physically blocked my exit, telling me he wouldn't let me in unless I was on my medication. I don't understand why he would take it on himself to treat people that way.

For whatever reason, the staff at the hostel gave me a sheet of paper with a calendar list of activities put on by the Schizophrenia Society. A volunteer came one day and drove me to one of the meetings. On this night, they had set up a group meeting for people with Schizophrenia to support each other. We started out going around the room introducing ourselves, and when it got to my turn to do so, I stood up and said, "My name is Doctor Gordon Mowat, and I research the disease of schizophrenia." No one even batted an eye to that. Personally, I believed it to be true. Later we went out for a break to have a cigarette, and this guy started talking to me about how he was working on a construction project to improve solar heating on houses, and he described it to me as if he was working on my house. The only home I had ever known was my dad's house in St. Albert, but his words caused me to become very confused and disoriented. Somehow as I was there talking to him, I had these ideas force their way into my head that I had my very own house and this guy was working for me.

The funny thing was that while I had hallucinatory thoughts and ideas, half of my mind knew they were false, but deep inside I wanted to tell everyone that I was some king or wealthy person, that I owned this and controlled all that. The delusions were that strong. While I was talking to another guy there, I had let it slip that I wanted to one day become Prime Minister of Canada. After saying this, a kind person, a fellow sufferer, started talking to me and tried to explain that he had delusionary thoughts like that at one time as well. He added that I was sick, and didn't need to set such impossible standards to feel okay about myself. It surprised me a lot that despite that I was obviously quite ill these people tried to help and support me. I remember I got a lot more out of that meeting than any of the religious or abstinence meetings, though there were things to be learned in those as well. I think what I needed most at that time was to be around people who were going through what I was; I needed someone to talk to who understood my condition.

For some reason, most of my delusional thinking seemed to focus on this one young woman who had never had anything to do with me. I still have invasive thoughts about her despite the medications that have worked well for me for many years now. She was a fellow student in my junior high and high school, but I was never even friends with her. She had gone out of her way a couple of times to be kind to me but, unfortunately, as time passed those kind words were simply fuel to my fire of madness.

As I look back at the web of messed up ideas and delusions, I can understand why mentally ill people are very often victims of abuse and assault. Although it seems funny for me to say this, not being a follower of the Freudian school of thought, schizophrenia and my type of bipolar disorder make the ego run wild in a sick person. Thoughts that find their way into your head tell you that you are the richest or the strongest or the smartest. The idea that you are sitting in a hospital or some crummy apartment doesn't even enter the equation, and no talking to or confrontation will convince you of the truth. What a lot of people don't completely realize is that medication is necessary, but you also need to make the person feel worthwhile, teach them how to manage their moods and thoughts and adjust to relationships and responsibilities just like anyone else.

In one of my earlier visits to the Alberta Hospital, I had a friend who would often say things to me that were extremely weird. I didn't mind at all because sometimes I thought them as well. I don't know why, but the staff would go out of their way to try and convince him that his delusions were false. This arguing and insulting seemed to be a useless effort. He would say things like, "I am everything at once." And you could see in his eyes that his mind was swimming in delusion and possibly a hallucination. I remember him saying that phrase because a couple of years later when I was trying to learn about religion and the Bible and all, it was hard for me to imagine Jesus without thinking of this poor guy I knew, who likely wondered at times if he was the real Son of God.

I have a clear memory of enjoying this guy's company. It helps in any situation to have a friend, but when locked up in a mental hospital it means even more. One time one of the ruder nurses said something to him about his Doctor wanting to see him, and he said, "I don't need to see the Doctor. He's in a coma." I don't know why but it seemed so funny at the time. He had this talent to state things that weren't exactly reality, but to use explosive words when he said them, like a talented poet.

I saw this guy later, and not only did he not know me, and I barely recognized him, but he had also changed immensely. I think his recovery from his poor state was due to one of the newer anti-psychotic medications known in some circles as "Personality drugs." The man appeared to be doing well; he didn't have that 'thousand-yard stare' he once did and seemed quite healthy and happy. I had tried one of these medications myself once and it caused me to sleep all day and not be able to function, so I had my doctor discontinue it. Not long after a massive lawsuit came out that proved the drug caused diabetes and thousands of psychiatric patients were paid a settlement. When I first had known this guy, he was very much in need of help. I was sad to hear that this medication which was so miraculous could have been so detrimental to people's health.

Just about every day while I was in the shelter/hostel, my parents would come and take me for a coffee and if I was lucky they would buy me a pack of cigarettes or some fries. Often I would hear people complaining that I was some rich kid who didn't belong there, and on more than one occasion, I was nearly assaulted or robbed. There was one guy who I had known from an earlier trip to Alberta Hospital, who was only about five feet tall, who walked up to me and shoved a ring case in my face. He opened it, and there was a diamond ring in it worth at least $1,000. He said, or I think he said, "Just think of this as a gift from a millionaire." It didn't make any sense at all, and plus he never gave it to me. In my delusion-prone mind, I imagined it was all a plot to get me to marry this wealthy, controlling woman who for whatever reason had the ability to monitor my thoughts.

Every small space even in the hostel seemed to have a camera. Even my thinking appeared to be broadcast all over the world, and the people on TV would react what went on in my head and comment. The scope of my paranoia at that time knew no bounds. I often wonder how that part of my illness came out back then. I did have some symptoms of schizophrenia, but my doctors had always told me my diagnosis was just bipolar disorder. There is, of course, a possibility that my illness affects me differently than others. I know that I do have my ups and downs, which explains the bipolar. At times, I have delusional thinking and paranoia, but rarely visual hallucinations. The other thing that makes me curious about a diagnosis of schizophrenia is that my medication stops my symptoms of psychosis, something that doesn't always happen with people with severe schizophrenia. What my medication doesn't stop is some of the personality defects that I developed over the years as coping mechanisms. If I don't watch myself I can get too eager to tell people things and talk too much and interrupt others. This can drive people away but is sometimes very hard to control. I also tend to stay up all night and take on huge tasks. When I was a teen I would often stay up watching TV all night and then at 6:00 am when all the good late night shows ended, I would think the best idea in the world would be to read the entire encyclopedia, but then end up fast asleep in an hour.

When I try and make people understand what it is like to be sick mentally like I was when I was in that shelter, I will often ask them if they had ever seen the movie, "12 Monkeys" with Brad Pitt and Bruce Willis. In that film, Brad Pitt is incredible in the way he portrays a person with schizophrenia; he has one line where he says, "Maybe these people have made a computer and fed into it all my thoughts and actions, and they can predict my every move with it." I am paraphrasing, but if a person can watch that and understand that somehow Mr. Pitt was dead-on in his acting abilities, they will understand to a small extent what mentally ill people go through.

I don't remember how long I was in that 'poor-house.' I was so drugged up it was a true challenge even to go and eat or walk down the hall to smoke. I was not only handicapped by my illness, but also the medications did a real job on me. Finally, one day my parents came and picked me up and could see that something serious was going to happen to me in short order. I had terrible influenza and was displaying such inconsistency of thought patterns that if they hadn't done something, I would end up in jail or a grave. They took me to the University Hospital and demanded a psychiatrist see me. If they hadn't intervened, I don't know if I would be here writing this today.

I was beaten at that point, physically, mentally and spiritually. The doctor on call did end up interviewing me, and the last thing he did was ask me a list of questions. At the end of them, I laughed and told the psychiatrist that he was a good hypnotist. Right away he admitted me to the hospital, and a metaphorical curtain came down separating my life before from my life to be. I now wanted help. I now wanted to be treated for my problems. It wasn't going to be the end of my recovery journey, but it was going to be a beginning of a long road of trial and error and future stability. I had made it across the Rockies one last time, and now I was home. It had cost me everything but my life to go on that trip, it had even cost me my sanity. I was about to start on a different journey, one that takes place in a person's mind, in their relationships and in a person's entire world view. Their way of looking at all those around them.

Chapter Three: Bridges Still Burning

Being in the Psychiatric Ward at the University of Alberta Hospital was much better than being in the shelter, however not quite as good as being in the North Vancouver Hospital. I hate to think that I have sampled every hospital from Edmonton to the coast, but such is the nature of my illness. I must admit the U of A Hospital treated me well. There was nothing but the best nurses and doctors and other staff there. While wandering around the ward, hoping to find something that could inspire me, I found a book there about a pilot who had pioneered the Canadian North and worked his way up the ranks in an airline. It was a man named Grant McConachie, and he had mostly grown up in Edmonton. While reading it, I longed to have flown in those days. It had only been a couple of months since I last took a flying lesson and my instructor had been strongly encouraging me to solo. In the time period of this pilot I read about, it only took about 30 hours of flying to get your Commercial Pilot's license, and I don't think there was even a very in-depth medical. Holding on to that idea in my head that I could somehow still be a pilot was detrimental to my recovery. Flying seemed to define who I was, though something greater was to come with time. I simply had no interest in other things than flying at the time. Planes and flight had claimed me, at least for a few years. As I look back though, it may have been a much better thing that I didn't pursue a career in flying. I liked it, but I get so much more meaning out of what I do now, which is to write and educate, mostly regarding mental health awareness. I recall as a teen delivering pizza I lamented that the job was contingent on me having a car. Later, in more physical work, I felt used because the job depended on my muscles. Being a person whow experienced life with mental illness, writing and speaking, and instructing classes of different types. I feel fulfillment, because my job rests on my knowledge, my interpersonal skills, and even to an extent my compassion.

I whiled away the first few days in the University Hospital reading about Grant and his death-defying stunts and how he always grabbed the bull by the horns when he did anything. The story gave me hope and inspiration when I was going through one of the hardest parts of my young life. Grant was a real bush pilot hero to look up to. An example of how he faced his problems happened once as he got older. At one point, he had some chest pains which turned out to be a heart problem. So, he went out and tried to get all the exercise possible in hopes of strengthening his heart, then found out from a doctor the thing for him to do was to have gotten all the rest he could and that his actions nearly killed him. I had been hearing about the tenacity of Canadian Pilots now for some time, and even though I never got my license, having gone through all the training hours and earning my Sergeant's stripes in Cadets made me feel a part of this tradition.

I feel strongly that my past in the Cadets and my training as a pilot may have been the only thing that got me through some of those tough times I went through after my return to Edmonton. Despite that I never did solo, I still felt it was worth it to spend all that money on flying and traveling two or three hours on the bus every day to the airport. It gave me an experience that few people have. Part of me was relieved that I wouldn't fly anymore after coming back. Instead of having dreams that I was a cold and callous person who would never find love, when I was flying I would have terrifying nightmares of flying a jumbo jet and being out of control and crashing, killing myself and everyone on board.

A couple of days after getting into the hospital, I phoned up the house of a young woman I had known from school. I knew her brother well, and her brother knew I cared about her. He answered the phone, and I asked to speak to Mrs. Chisolm, and he gave the phone to his sister. It was a bit of a shock hearing her voice, but I told her I wanted to talk to her mom. I tried to apologize for an incident that had happened earlier that year where I had gone to their house and walked in the door without permission and tried to explain that I had a mental illness and was in the hospital and was trying to get my life in order and take responsibility for my actions. She was forgiving and nice about it, considering her husband seemed to have wanted to put me in the electric chair when the incident happened. I hung up, a few days later my mom told me someone had called for me, and she offered the person my number but she didn't take it. I still wonder if that had been my last chance at being on that young woman's good side or if it was the other young woman that had changed her number and wouldn't answer my letters. Either way, I realized that coming back to Edmonton was not going to be what I had hoped it would be. I was going to be on my own and would have to start my life and my relationships from the ground up. It astounds me now when I look back and it seems all my memories were strung together stories of women I had crushes on, but never had any kind of deep relationships with. It makes me wonder how much of an egotist I was, claiming that I cared for one girl asking her out and then just moving on to hit on the next one. I constantly needed to feed my low self-esteem with compliments and indications that others found me attractive. I suppose it may have stemmed from being insulted, teased, and bullied at an earlier age. Either way, it was going to have to stop soon. Looks or not, unless I did some serious maturing, I would never know the dream I had of being a parent and having someone to care about.

One of the other things I did while I was in the U of A hospital was to attend a church service. I had been thinking about when I was in high school and driving into the student parking lot when things would get weird and thoughts of Armageddon would come to me. I would get these strange feelings that the world was going to end and I knew that people who went to church had a better grasp on this idea than I did. They knew something that was a comfort to them that helped them to get through. I never saw myself as a bad person, but I had a lot of traits that indicated I had little moral grounding. I smoked and I drank. At times, I had tried pot and hash and I often swore like a trucker saying negative things about women whenever I thought I could get away with it.

All my life I had been deathly afraid of nuclear war and greatly feared the thought that not only would I die in it, but all my family and friends and everyone I ever knew would die in it. Church seemed to offer a solution to my fear, that if I went, and did what they told me, I would live on in heaven and hopefully so would the people I cared about. This fear was one of the key elements of my abnormal behavior, going as far back as my younger days camping with my family, training myself to survive in the wild. The effect of these thoughts of end times was the main reason that my parents put me in the hospital back when I was 14. I had been obsessed with weapons and bombs, I wore army combat clothes all the time and there was even a morning when the roof kept cracking from a change in temperature and I went to my dad fearful that Russian paratroopers were landing on our house.

After I had attended the service in the hospital, I talked to the pastor, and I asked him if the Bible talked about things that were happening in the world in politics and about the end of the world. He plainly told me that there is some stuff in the Bible about all that but not to worry about it. He gave me a New Testament and sent me on my way. I didn't know how to take what he had said to me.

Along with the news that I was now on my own, failing miserably at my early attempts of romance, while in the hospital I got word that my Aunt Joanne had killed herself through an overdose of medications. She and my Uncle Ted had lived in the same apartment complex, and I hadn't spoken to them in years. I didn't remember all that much about my Aunt. One time when we were down in Drumheller for a family event, she was there. I sat while she talked for half an hour but didn't pay attention. I couldn't tell you a single word she said, although I do remember that afterward, she told my dad that she had given us kids the 'birds and the bees' speech. I think that angered my Dad, but for me, it went right past. It's amazing how kids can just tune some things out. I had always known her to be a bit odd but over the years occasionally I tried to get my Mom to call her up but she wouldn't. When I was in Alberta Hospital when I was 18, she was in a ward just across the hall, but we never spoke in the three months I was there. It was sad to think, as I had heard later from my Uncle, that she was in the deepest stages of depression. Although mental illness is not 100% guaranteed hereditary, on my mother's side of the family mental illness has effected just about all of us from my cousins to my mom's grandmother.

While I was on the psychiatric ward, I had long since run out of cigarettes. It had taken all my money to pay back rent and front rent in the Traveler's Hostel I lived in, plus paying for my ticket to Edmonton. For a while, I smoked a pipe with pipe tobacco and then that ran out, so I removed the tobacco from butts in the ashtray and put it in my pipe. I learned years later that people who have mental illnesses have a neurotransmitter that their medications inhibit and cigarette smoking also inhibits this chemical in similar ways. Hence, it is detrimental to a person with a mental health condition to not have nicotine or a nicotine replacement like patches or gum. It got to the point where one of the nurses confronted my dad and just about demanded he buy me some cigarettes. He ended up giving me a carton or two that he found in my Aunt's apartment. It was a nice gesture, but I felt very hurt that I had grown so far apart from all my family members at that time in my life when I needed their support and love more than ever. My sister even lived right across the street from the hospital and never came to visit. The depths of my loneliness and isolation knew no bounds.

Feeding my spiritual needs and my love of history, I picked up another book that I found on the ward about miracles that happened during World War Two. It was fascinating, reading about my favorite time in history and the stories being all about proof of the existence of God. What I had seen of church and religion seemed to offer me a solution to the lack of love in my life, my lack of purpose, and my lack of understanding of the world around me. I wanted to find a place to worship but I knew very little about any type of church. The 'Miracles' book left me with a lot of questions in my head, and it would take years before I could find answers.

One of the things I ended up doing was attend an anonymous meeting like the ones I had gone to before that were held in the hospital. At the meeting, I met a very kind and man of about 50 who took me under his wing. His name was John, and he had been to the lowest and highest places a person could go. I want to do him justice and of course speak well of him, but the meetings are supposed to be anonymous. He had a lot of wisdom to share with me, but sadly, he is long since passed away. After meeting him, I started attending more meetings and meeting people associated with the organization. It helped to while away the long and tedious hours that come with any hospital admission. Not too long later I was told to get ready to leave the hospital, and John planned for me to move into a small room in his house.

Over the next couple of months, I would take the bus to my appointments; I made an application to start school, and I also made long-term plans to attend Journalism School at what was then Grant MacEwan Community College (now a University). Each day I would get up and eat, pace around or go to the grocery store. My new landlord John had a nephew that lived in the house and sometimes we would go for coffee or walk up to the arcade. Upstairs there was a guy who worked as a security guard and got me a job in the field I was to work in for 15 of the next 20 years.

I appreciated the way the people there treated me with extraordinary kindness. I can't forget when, because of the effects of my medications, my hands used to shake so bad I couldn't write legibly. So, my security guard friend who lived upstairs filled out my job applications. John also had his ex-wife living in that house, and she had mental health issues like mine. One time we were sitting out in the garden in the back and out of nowhere, she said to me, "Would you like five dollars?" Normally I would have refused, but times were tough then, and five dollars went a long way, so I took it and greatly appreciated it.

I remember having lost any sense of hope while I was living there. My life was simple, I would get up, have a coffee, walk to a bookstore and buy a comic book, then stop in at the arcade. A few nights a week John would drive me to a meeting and I would drink far too much coffee. Depression and desperation were serious issues for me. But then one day out of nowhere I was watching a PBS special TV show that was a live performance of Neil Young. It all seemed to be just an ordinary concert, but then he sang a song called "Heart of Gold" and somehow it seemed to speak directly to my heart. I still play the song now and then when I feel bad, which is rare, but at the time it was like Neil Young had reached down right into my soul and found something worthwhile and beautiful about me as a human being. It seemed like right at that point my mental health began to improve and I didn't feel so bad about who I was anymore.

There were some bad times there as well, once John came up and yelled at me and said I needed a shower because I stank. He was right, though. Typically, I took a hot, relaxing bath every day, but there was no tub in my part of the property it was so cold in that house. To top it off, I wasn't used to the temperature difference between Vancouver and Edmonton, which made showering difficult. Another time John came up to me and said, "Oh yeah, I went in and cleaned your room for you. You should thank me."

"You're not allowed in my room without my permission," I said with more than a little shock in my voice.

"It's my house. I can do whatever I want." It was his house, but since when do you rent something out and retain full use of it?

I don't know why the situation has gotten so bad, but until I moved into government-approved housing I never have in my 27 years of living on my own had a landlord who followed the set written laws governing housing (The Landlord and Tenant Act). I feel this is important because many people who get kicked out have no defense against unscrupulous landlords and a lot of those who are homeless in Edmonton are also mentally ill. Ignoring the law and people's rights (and not enforcing these laws) leads to deaths and social problems that aren't going to go away.

I don't blame John because he went in and cleaned my room, although I did hear that not long after someone took him to task on how he was treating his renters. He stayed my friend for a long time. Years later he and his mentally ill ex-wife passed away. I spoke to a friend of theirs, and he told me in the last days before they died, the two of them re-married and I thought it was such a beautiful thing. He had a heart of gold, and so did his now-in-Heaven wife.

Chapter Four: New High School for Older Students

I moved out to a new place near the school I wanted to go to and the next few months seemed to take forever as I waited all alone in my small apartment for school to start. Life in the inner city of Edmonton was so far removed from life in Vancouver or St. Albert. I just didn't seem to meet anyone my age, and so when I ran into an old friend I had known for years, I quickly consented to go to church with him in the hopes that we could go back to being good friends like when we were kids. It was a strange experience because I still had quite a bit of the rebellious youth side of me and sometimes I would argue with people over what their beliefs were. It was so confusing to see my friend's dad (who I thought was a pretty intelligent and likable guy) practically order me not to question the Bible. I started to understand more of how my friend's upbringing had gone and why he was a little funny in some ways. Rules everywhere about everything, and intolerance for any other viewpoint.

I passed the days by going to my friend's house, where we would drink iced tea and play cards, I would read the Bible with him and sometimes we would play pool at the local arcade. I was so destitute at that time it was hard for me to come up with the 50 cents it took to play a game of pool but when I did, I enjoyed myself. Growing up there was nothing I liked more than a game of eight-ball. The sad thing was that though it was fun, John once explained to me that being good at pool is not a useful skill. When I think back now, I had dollar signs in my eyes, hoping to get good enough to gamble and enter tournaments like in the movies. I loved to play pool and at one point in my life had thought about becoming a professional but as I have grown, I only see the bad places a life choice like that would have taken me. I haven't played in years.

When school finally did start up, I felt so good to have a place to go, things to do. I started a whole new life but still I had to take my medications and visit my Doctors every week or two. It became harder and harder for me to keep up with my schoolwork because the doctors had put me on a drug called Lithium, and it made my hands shake like I was a 90-year-old man. It was terribly embarrassing, and soon I made the unfortunate decision to go off the drug. I remember I had felt like this school year was going to be my last chance ever to make something of myself, ever be anyone of any significance. Plans and even funding were in place for me to take a 2-year Journalism course, maybe even apply to a prestigious program in Quebec. Writing was my biggest dream back then.

I can remember that one of the few things I had done that meant anything to me that year was to save up what little I had to buy an electric typewriter. I started out just keeping a journal, trying to fill a page a day and then I would scour the library and any place I could to get a deal for poetry books to read. I even wrote a few short stories that I eventually adapted into my first book, "Through the Withering Storm." Little did I know that this would one day be my life's work.

One of my favorite classes at my new school was Biology. We had this great teacher who was a bit old and dressed in fashions that died in the 1970s, but he was a fun teacher to have. He went by the name of 'Dick,' and everyone liked him a lot. He would go into detail about things that most teachers never bothered telling students. One thing I recall was him telling us about a teacher who had told a class in California that every species of creature was named and classified. The class took this as a challenge, he said, and they went out into the desert with lights and special cameras and found several new ones. He made people forget that they were in a run-down school for second chances.

Dick was an odd person in some ways, but a kind and friendly one. He was a smoker and was always ready to lend one out with a smile when you caught him smoking outside. In his class was the girl who was to become the love of my life, I will call her Debbie. One of the things he would always tell us at the end of class was for us to go home and read a 'sexy' book—he meant our biology text of course.

I remember seeing that girl in the class every day; she was so lovely. Her blond hair was in a ponytail, her brown Native Indian leather jacket adorned with tassels fitting her slim but shapely figure so well. A few times I saw her in the hall, her nose deep in a book and I thought it was just the sexiest thing in the world that she seemed to love literature like I did. One day I went out to smoke, and there she was. I started talking to her about our class and our teacher and before I knew it we were best friends.

It wasn't long before Debbie and I were studying together and going to the mall together, out to eat or for coffee all the time. One of the things we loved doing was going to a bar near my apartment and drinking coffee and watching their big screen TV with the American music video channel on. There was so much good music out then, Debbie got me interested in Leonard Cohen, who had just put out a killer album called "The Future" and we would sit and watch Nirvana and the Tragically Hip until Debbie had to take the late bus home. She was so sweet to me, doing things like making coffee and bringing it for me to try in a thermos from home. The only bad thing about her was that she was living with her boyfriend, and I felt horrible about it because I had a feeling she was falling in love with me and that I was with her. I even had a talk with him one night offering to back down and get out of their lives, but he said I didn't have to. I wonder what might have happened to my life if I had done that.

One day the bunch of us went out and had quite a few drinks and then went back to Debbie's place and her boyfriend went into their bedroom to fall asleep. Debbie sat there on her couch and looked at me through her intoxicated eyes and no matter what I would say or do she would snuggle up beside me and look deep into my eyes. Finally, she told me what I had known. Debbie told me about her deep feelings for me, but I said there was no way I would have a relationship with her until she left her boyfriend. She seemed to accept this and then it was time for me to catch the first bus and so she walked me there. We stopped on our way, hidden from prying eyes and she gave me the deepest, wettest most passionate kiss I had ever had up to that point in my young life. I took the bus home and had a hard time sleeping; I didn't know what was going to happen. I didn't even know if I would see her again. By that time, I had written my midterm exams and took my few diploma credits and quit school. All I was living for was to hang out with her.

The next day Debbie came over to my apartment and started off where we had stopped the night before. We talked for a while, and somehow I maneuvered myself close to her, and we started kissing. It wasn't any necking like I had done before, which was two people trying to get off on each other. To me, it seemed like some magical expression of mutual love. All of it was so new to me, not only had I never got as far with a woman like this before, I had never cared like this about someone who felt the same way about me before. I remember in one of the many books I used to read about aviation that flying a plane was the most fun you could have outside the bedroom. When I connected with Debbie like this and we both had strong feelings for each other, I understood what that meant and for the first time in my life didn't feel so bad that I would never be a pilot again. We ended up in my bedroom but stopped before the final act. I wanted to complete the act of lovemaking with her, but she stopped me because we had no protection.

The next day she came over again, and I didn't know what to say to her. I wanted her to break up with her boyfriend but for some reason, she just let things happen and waited for him to find out. I blame myself for not showing her enough how I felt, how important she was to me. Maybe if I had she would have taken that huge step for me. When Debbie got to my apartment on that second day, she smiled at me and took a condom out of her purse. That first time with her that followed was better than anything I had ever experienced. Now, many years later, she told me she didn't remember much about our experiences together except that after that I had this weird, kind of angry look about me afterwards.

We went on like this for a few weeks. Debbie's boyfriend came to confront us and she finally told him what was going on. She kicked him out of her apartment and then moved into a new place and I kept my one bedroom. In the odd moments when we weren't doing anything together, I would read this book that had my full attention: James A. Michener's "Space," which was his interpretation of the entire Space Program in the US from its beginnings until a few years into the future. As I find with any of Michener's works I pick up, it was a book that changed the way I looked at a lot of things. Despite that I was technically disabled due to my illness and the need for medications, I was still passionately fascinated with the space program.

After all we went through, Debbie decided to go back to her ex-boyfriend. On the last day I was to stay over, and the last day we were to be a couple, Debbie and I went to a popular west end bar. I started a conversation with a young woman sitting beside me and Debbie kind of plastered herself all over some other guy. The lounge was much too noisy to chat, so the girl I met and I wrote on paper and napkins back and forth, and I think we ended up exchanging phone numbers. Debbie ended up getting blasted out of her mind at some party we went to, and after the host of the party threatened me for getting angry with her, I managed to get out in one piece and take Debbie home.

The young woman I met at the bar, was named Krista and she sort of filled the hole that Debbie had left in my life, though it was a terribly painful break-up, perhaps made worse by the fact that Debbie didn't seem to care at all since she had a backup boyfriend. I often wish that I had taken more time to form a relationship with Debbie that would have lasted us more than two months. My emotions were fragile and I let myself fall hard for her. Some of the best advice I had gotten from people I went to church with was that "a condom can't heal a broken heart."

Krista was impressive. She was a bit heavy but attractive and had a great sense of humor. I remember looking at her bus pass, and on it there was a line saying, "In case of emergency, contact:" and she had written, "The Police Stupid!" She would do the weirdest things sometimes. I remember being in a mall with her and though I knew she had no money, she went to a burger joint and came back and handed me a cheeseburger. Soon she was to reveal to me a secret that I didn't want to hear. In fact, to this day, I don't even know if it was true or not. She told me that she was working for a guy who did seriously evil things. Krista went on to say he had wanted to know more about me but she wouldn't let him 'recruit me' because she was in love with me. I think Krista was the first female I knew who took me for a ride like those other possible sociopaths had done.

One night I called her up and talked to her for a few minutes, and as I was about to hang up the phone, she whispered: "Help me." Into the phone. I called the Police, and they went down in a hurry and kicked out a person that was in her apartment. Krista said he had tried to rape her, and the next day I saw her she had a black eye. She told me she had been beaten up by someone in the mall because she had been defending my actions. It was so hard to keep up with her. It seemed everything was a lie but her black eye was real.

Around that time, I had my eye on an old Apple IIe computer I wanted to use for typing up my stories and poems and playing video games. I had a hard time finding work but eventually found a job at a car wash. There I would toil and labor eight to ten hours a day, and because of how they only let employees punch in while they were working on cars, I would get 4 hours pay a day if I was lucky. It was a pretty brutal environment; the supervisor would slam things around and yell at people. The money was a pittance. Still, I was soon able to buy my first computer and had endless fun with it. The main problem was that it didn't have a word processing program or a printer, but I was thrilled to have my own computer at the time nonetheless. I even made friends with and hung around with some cool people who worked there and often came to my house to hang out.

Krista dropped out of the picture not long after that. I just couldn't take her lying and manipulating. For reasons that escape me, I got to know a young woman who was pregnant and a bit messed up. She had previously been a prostitute and been tested and found to be HIV negative. I longed for any human contact, so we had one night together. The next day I called her, and she said she had just found a new boyfriend who was a drug dealer. A week or so down the road she called me up asking if a friend of hers could stay over at my place.

Saying yes to that was the worst mistake I could have ever made. This guy not only decided to come over, he decided to move in, and he kept bringing more and more friends over, filling my apartment with street people. In the two or three months he was there, he never paid a cent of rent and neither did any of his friends. Not paying rent might not have been so bad, but he ran my phone bill up to over $800, and when I tried to explain to him that this was his responsibility he looked over the bill and denied making any of the calls. When I finally got rid of him, he and his cronies took anything that wasn't nailed down and kept my keys.

The big thing that bothered me about all that was that they kept one of my six volumes of the complete works of William Shakespeare which had been a gift from my parents when I was 16. That was a time when I couldn't get enough poetry and philosophy from books. Their next stop was an apartment downstairs from me, which, in a few short weeks, was condemned by the health authority. I went back to my incredibly lonely existence in that small place, hoping that soon going to Journalism School would be my salvation from all this.

While I was working at the car wash, I walked into work one day and saw a picture of a guy I knew well right on the front page of the newspaper, with the headline, "Murdered." I grabbed the paper and learned that something had happened overseas that would bring an end for many years to the positive light the military enjoyed among the Canadian public. The government had sent the former Airborne Regiment to Somalia, and in the past couple of days, someone had brought to light a lot of negative things. I was to learn later that the man I knew had been the first one to try and take the injustices to the authorities. Sadly, because of a dual factor of playing a small part in the killing and the fact that the person who was mostly to blame was mentally unfit to stand trial, my friend was scapegoated. Soon after I made the money I needed and bought my computer, my friend came to visit me while he was on trial. I wanted to help him in any way I could, but there was nothing I could do for him. I even failed at being his friend because my illness returned in full force at the exact time he came to visit.

We did a few things together, I offered to help him write a book about the incident, but my mental health was declining fast. That was when I did one of those things that I run through in my head over and over. For whatever reason, paranoia, fear, delusion-it could have been anything: I stole from the one friend I had in this world. My mind was full of delusional fear, I was slowly starving in that place, and something told me it would be okay. Against any decency left in me, I took $100 out of his wallet, and he would never forgive me. A few years later, when he was out of prison, I gave a mutual friend $50 to give to him with a promise of full repayment, but he brought back the message that the friendship was over for good.

Shortly after my friend left, my dad called me and asked me to come along with him to take my mom to the hospital. I was on the jagged edge at this point, at least as bad off as when I had first gone to the hospital. My mom also spoke to me, and I remember her saying, "Leify, I need you!" Words to which only a cold-hearted devil could say no. When my Dad, Brother, and

Mom came, I tried to get in the car, but I got into an argument with my Dad and Brother about what needed to be done. After a shouting match, I finally got in the car, and on to the hospital we went.

This trip to the hospital was yet another thing that happened that I feel horrible about. We got to there and my mom was in tears wanting to get help but her Doctor wanted me to take her place in the Psychiatric wing. I complied, feeling a bit happy that I didn't have to be beaten up or questioned by the Police to get the help that was needed this time and consented. I ended up in the locked ward of the Grey Nuns Hospital, and there I would stay for the rest of the summer. When I think back to that day, I often wonder how I could have been so cold as to take my Mom's spot, but I also understand that it was more up to my Dad than me, who had most likely told the doctor about what had been going on with me in the past while. It was a scary thing; I had become extremely paranoid and delusional. I thought that there were cameras and listening devices all around, even when I went to take out the garbage I thought I was being filmed and that someone was going to go through my garbage. There was no escape from that hell of false ideas. It had all started one night when I was on my computer and suddenly felt that I could type questions into the keyboard and people on the radio would answer them. In a way, I had thought if I isolated myself in that small apartment that voices and delusions wouldn't reach me, but still they found a way into my head.

When they first admitted me to that Hospital, I spent quite a bit of time in a sterile, unfriendly, locked psychiatric ward, hanging around in pajamas and trying to entertain myself as best I could, smoking, doing puzzles out of the paper, eating and watching TV. I made one call to Debbie and tried to tell her that I loved her and she said to me, "So, what do you want me to do about it?" She didn't even want to visit. I called up the Youth Pastor of the church I was attending and asked if he could get someone to visit me and he told me, "Well, there's nothing I can do. Whose fault is it you're in there?" As though I had been in a car accident and because the injury was my fault he couldn't acknowledge that I was in pain. I like to think the injury wasn't my fault but I was the one who had strayed from the care of my psychiatrist months before. But it seemed it was almost like I had committed a crime and he had already convicted me of it. I wonder in what part of the criminal code the law exists that it is illegal to be confused and delusional and I would also like to know where it says, "guilty until proven innocent." It just seemed wrong that a pastor would seem to have no compassion for what I was going through.

The days slipped by and eventually they gave me back my regular clothing, which they said meant they would transfer me soon to one of the open wards. Then for some reason, I didn't do something the way a nurse felt I should, and she called security to hold me down and give me an injection. They also wanted to lock me in my room and take my clothes away. At that time, I didn't have a high opinion of those injections, and I liked the idea less of being forced to do something. So, when the security guards came, rather than being stripped bare in front of a ticked off nurse by two bodybuilders, both much bigger than me, I told them I was willing to go in my room, and that they could see for themselves I wasn't all agitated or violent. But if they tried to hold me down for that injection they would have a real fight on their hands. The nurse was livid, but it was the security guards who were the ones who would have had to do the rough work, so they agreed. They went into my room, put the mattress on the floor and took my bed out of it.

I hated the idea that anyone on a psychiatric ward could just decide you needed an injection and an isolation order. Isolation, even for someone who is used to it is such a cruel punishment. I have often felt that there should be a process where they need a doctor's order or two nurses to sign off on an isolation order. Because of feeling this way, when they decided I could come out of my room, I had a surprise for them. First I refused to put my mattress back on my bed and second I refused to eat out of protest. I don't know if any of them had dealt with this sort of thing before because it seemed to throw them for a loop. There was even one Doctor who had nothing to do with my case that came up to me and tried to give me a lecture on how he felt about my attitude. I ended up giving him a lecture on how people in hospitals are human beings and heard no more of it from him.

After a longer than normal stretch of time, they put me in one of the open wards, and my mom was in the ward as well by that time. I started to comply with treatment, but for some reason, doctors don't always know how a medication will work for someone until they try it. It reminds me of what doctors in World War One would have to do when there was no X-Ray machine available, and someone had shrapnel or a bullet lodged inside of them. They simply had to keep stabbing the area with a scalpel until they had located the foreign object, and I would suppose leave quite a scar. With my psychiatrist, he decided to try me out on a medication that helped my mood swings and delusional thinking, but left me restless and edgy to the point where I couldn't stand still or sit for any length of time. It was horrible, but I wanted to go home so bad I didn't ask for a medication change. There is a lot of hope coming with new discoveries and treatments now; there are active MRI machines and other diagnostic tools that could one day make psychiatry a lot more of an exact science, just like in World War One when portable X-ray machines were developed. I think though, that it will take a lot of voices and a lot of conversations to bring to light some of the more unfortunate and cruel aspects of modern psychiatric treatment.

On the last day I was supposed to be in the hospital; there was a young kid who was joking around with me, and I chased him around a sofa for fun. Unfortunately, I tripped on the carpet and in the fall, broke my hand. The doctor decided to keep me there an extra couple of days to settle down, and when I saw the kid next, he was pointing at me, proudly saying he had broken my hand. I grabbed him with my cast hand and gave him a couple of good slaps, and then went back to my room. Another uproar came up because of this, and despite that this kid was the worst behaved person on the ward, the staff threatened me from all sides with assault charges and so on. They weren't even hard slaps. I just wanted to let this kid know that causing someone extreme pain and injury isn't something to be proud of. Looking back, a lot of my behavior in that hospital, and before I went in there were acts of violence based on ignorance, misunderstanding and an immature lack of self-control. This was something I needed to grow out of, this was something that would keep on getting in the way of my recovery. As a young person who was the victim of violence on many occasions, I swore I would never end up the bully or the criminal that went along with a violent attitude, but it seemed I had been pushed to extremes and had forgotten the things I once held dear. I like to think that now I have grown past all that as I moved more fully into recovery. All it took was to develop a sense of compassion and understanding about others that I learned through counselling, maturing, and meditation. I still have my edgy days, but looking at the world through the eyes of others has helped me immensely to become more of a peaceful and accepting person.

Somehow my sharp tongue saved me from being in the hospital longer once again, and I left the hospital as summer ended. Just before I got there, Grant McEwan Community College had given me notice that though they accepted me, the Journalism program had been canceled. I was now facing a long cold winter with little to do, in total isolation on a medication that was intolerable. Even my computer offered me little solace.

The next weeks were all made up of dark days. I loved to read. It was often the only thing that kept me going, but I was so restless from my medication that I just could not sit still. I have this rule I made for myself that no matter how difficult it is, no matter what the situation, I try and move forward in my knowledge or skills each day, and thus, my life has gotten better over the years and I haven't had the feeling of wasting time.

As a young child, I wasted so much time in front of the TV and I regretted it. On my release from the hospital, I wanted to keep reading, keep learning. So, I found a book of short stories and I forced myself through them, usually just being able to finish one a day. I saw my doctor in far off Millwoods a few times; then I tried going back to the University Hospital and ended up seeing a very compassionate and intelligent Psychiatrist. I begged him to find an alternative to the medication I was taking. He found something for me, something that was experimental for people with bipolar disorder, something that had caused cataracts in dogs and sometimes made people's hair fall out, but I took it, and it caused a real turning point in my life. There was just one bad side effect to the drug. It caused me diarrhea, but it helped a great deal, and I was soon able to do more things like reading although I was in a sort of blue funk of depression. Soon, I found another security job that didn't pay too badly. For the most part, until a time far in the future that I lowered my dose without permission, I was not to have problems with mania again. I had been through a lot, and there was a lot I would go through until I could call myself truly 'well' again. All I had was a medication that seemed to work on my symptoms and a fresh chance at having a life outside of a hospital.

Chapter Five: Broken Hearts and Summer Romance

The new medication seemed to work well for me, but I felt I lacked one important thing: a newer computer with a word processor and printer so I could write and edit my growing stack of stories. I also wanted a lot of other stuff that people with actual jobs had, like a motorbike and a car and all the toys that grown men conveniently allow themselves. I sat down one day and wrote out everything my heart desired, from a motorcycle to a brand-new computer, and funny enough, in ten years I sat down to this same list and looked at what I had, and realized I had accomplished all of it. This phenomenon speaks volumes about the power of goal-setting, though I was to go through some pretty lean times first. I like to think that going through those hard times has taught me how to negotiate for deals, how to sell and how to run a business; skills that have made my writing life a success even though I am nowhere near the big time.

Something I don't like to talk about much is a young woman named Nancy I dated on a couple of occasions while in high school. I had met her at a summer camp. She was attractive and intelligent, and had an incredible sense of humor. A few months after we first got together in Edmonton after camp, I stopped calling her, and she never called me back. So, I just let the whole thing go. I think it was a self-esteem issue that would cause me to punish myself by just shutting things out of my life that had the potential to make me happy. It was almost like I wanted people to pity me, or go out of their way to connect with me, when it was a poor way to try and communicate pain, and a desire for someone to care about me. Despite that I hadn't seen Nancy in years, I never seemed to be able to stop thinking about her. The summer camp we met at was a two-part course put on by the Alberta Government for youth leaders, and I remember it as being one of the best and most enlightening parts of my life to that point. We went canoeing, rock face climbing, had classes in leadership, teaching, etc. The staff was fantastic, and they taught us all a lot of self-awareness concepts and life skills. There were a few girls there, but I was knocked flat by just one of them. I often wish she had never seen the darker side of my mental illness, but she did years later.

Nancy was a kids' youth leader at a YMCA summer camp and I was there as an Air Cadet. Her job as a YMCA counsellor was to teach kids different things that would hopefully prepare them for life. She seemed to have such a limitless capacity for caring. It was almost as if she had the things I lacked and desperately wished I could have. There was something I could see in her eyes: the love for all things maybe, and the ability to nurture and love children not even her own.

After that summer when I went back to school, I was in a pattern of staying up all night, sleeping just a couple of hours before school, and then **after** I had finished my classes for the day, going for a nap. During these nap times, I would have the worst possible dreams. They were dreams that I was a cold and cruel person and that people-especially children-didn't like me. I feared that I would one day die single, a monster with a military mindset having never experienced love between myself and a woman, or love between father and child. All the while I was cursing myself for not being a compassionate being like Nancy was. As time passed, I slipped deeper and deeper into a self-destructive depression, and as I look back now, I wonder if I was laying the groundwork for a severe delusional psychosis. Years later I had called Nancy from Vancouver, and we were friends again for a short while at a time when my mental health was rapidly declining. My flawed brain took on the idea that she cared deeply for me and wanted to marry me and she soon severed all contact with me.

How this relates to my adult years was that when I was just past 21, I was attending a Pentecostal church down the street from my apartment. I was much less depressed then, I also liked the way they would lay down moral guidelines and rules for living based on the Bible. I grew so much in the times I went there. I became a more caring, giving and honest person, but the journey towards who I am now was far from over. One evening, I stumbled across the opportunity to develop the side of me that I felt was gone forever with my teen years.

At church, a man got up and asked for people to volunteer to staff a children's camp he was organizing. I met with him, and after a couple of interviews, a police check and a promise that I wouldn't smoke in front of the children, he agreed to take me on as a camp counselor.

Going to that camp was one of the most magical experiences of my life. I met a lot of people my age, and I got to know these incredible young kids, all about ten years old. We would swim and play games and go horseback riding. I was destitute, and my parents were even worse off, but at this camp, I didn't mind at all. I had more than I needed of everything and I experienced an almost pure happiness. For the first time in my adult life, it didn't matter that I had this horrible illness boiling up under the surface of my conscious mind. I just had to care for and help these kids, and it was something I found that I loved doing.

There was a couple of young women at the camp and we became friends. I was starting to forget all about the problems, the bills, the depression and other things that I had left back home. In a way, I kind of wish I could have stayed at a camp like that forever.

One night I met up with a girl whose camp name was Mustang and her best friend, and we walked a long way out of camp and laid down in a ditch and stargazed and talked for a long time. This experience was all that I used to dream of; having female companionship, living far away from any town, being able to see all the billions of stars, spending time with kids, teaching them and having them look up to me. In all my dreams, I couldn't ask for more. When the camp ended, my self-destructive, cold heart told me I should decline to give out my address for the list they published with everyone's contact information and thus never saw 99% of those people again. For a while I cherished a postcard a little camper had given me, written to Bart, which was my camp name. It read: "Bart-thanks you!"

My roommate after I got home from that camp was a guy named Jeff. He had a few characteristics to him that were annoying. I had known Jeff and his sister from the Pentecostal church I attended at that time. Jeff had come into the church after living a life of literally being a mall rat, living on whatever couch or floor he could find and stealing to survive. Even though he was helping with rent, it wasn't worth it to have him there. Jeff had a theory that it was okay to lie to people if your end goal is to lead them to religion. He would come up with stories that he had been a black priest and that he was an officer in the military and a host of other things that I was sure weren't true.

I knew another guy, Dunzel, from the U of A Hospital psychiatric ward who didn't live too far from me. He had gotten the idea that he could save money if he moved in with a guy named Kevin down the hall from me when I was in my first apartment. Kevin was, by self-admission, an idiot. Kevin often tried to scare people by telling stories of eating human babies in dark rituals and being locked up in a mental hospital in a strait jacket and being fed through a tube for six months. Dunzel, despite my advice to the contrary, moved in with him and then when it didn't work out he kept trying to come over and sleep on the floor in my living room. I tried to stop him from doing it but then he would convince Jeff to allow him, and I had to deal with him lying on the floor of my apartment every morning. It was a total gong-show, but I often think I should have had a little more compassion. It was something that had often been shown to me by many people as I struggled to live alone with a mental illness and Dunzel had some serious problems.

The reason I moved out of my old building, was that there was a caretaker put in charge who was a complete ass. I always paid my rent; I was quiet, and I tried to get along with the other people in the building. Despite that, this caretaker took it upon himself to tell my dad that I was in with the wrong crowd and other things he didn't need to say to him, especially since I had gotten rid of all of them and didn't do any of the illegal or immoral things they did. One day not long after that, I saw him in the hall and told him not to talk to my parents because I didn't want them to worry about me. The things he was saying just scared my mom out of her wits. She was a sensitive and caring person, and all this talk only gave her more anxiety. I got mad and walked up to him, and told him to stop telling my parents anything, and we ended up in a verbal battle. It was time to leave that slimy place, but in my search to have friends and go to a church where I could feel nurtured and connected to a loving God, I would get into more trouble further down the road.

Even in a run-down, poorly managed apartment building like that, there were good people. Sometimes I would go over to Kevin's for pasta or video games. There was also another guy who used to buy bread for everyone in the building and pass it out free. People like that made living there tolerable.

Kevin had become the caretaker after the heavy-set, abusive, and manipulating guy left. The other caretaker had evicted me, and I desperately wanted out of that building, so I left without disputing it. I got most of my stuff out, but when I went back to get the rest Kevin had kicked in the door and stolen everything, including most of a $5,000 comic collection. It seemed that no matter where I lived, I would run into these people who stepped all over my rights and out and out stole from me, but there was no way to get the police to do anything about it. Often when I needed to call the police while living in that place, they would come down, explain how they couldn't or wouldn't do anything, and suggest that I move to the University area. I had a self-righteous idea that I could make a change in that neighborhood, plus the church I went to was only a few blocks away. The fact is, though, that police can't act as someone's private security force. They must pick their battles just like anyone else, and they had long since given up on the neighborhood, and the building where I lived.

So, I moved into a large apartment with Jeff and ended up feeling good about myself, thinking I had moved away from my problems, but soon realized that to do that I would have to do a lot more than change my address. A friend reminded me at the time that you can search the world for happiness and find it between your ears. I would add to that and say that I could run from my problems but I had to take my delusional, paranoid, depression-prone brain with me.

One day in my new place I was sitting down for lunch, and a guy came up to my window and offered me $20 to help him bring an apartment washer/dryer unit up to his apartment. I agreed and ended up getting to know the guy. He was gay and was living with HIV, back before people's lives could be significantly extended when they had HIV. He was a young man who was soon going to die.

His name was Don, and despite all the things going against him, he had a keen business sense, and was essentially a good person and a good friend. We got along well, I would visit sometimes and we would watch

TV and he would let me use his computer. Even though I'm not gay, I found that being around marginalized people of any type who are 'different' helps me a lot because there is a certain level of acceptance among people with chronic mental or physical health issues (not to say being gay is a mental illness). He and I would often drive up and down back alleys, looking for cars that were in good shape, but that had expired license plates. He would buy them dirt cheap and get them running and resell them for a decent profit. Those were good times. I don't think I ever made much money off Don, but I learned a fair bit about negotiating and looking for deals. There were only two things that concerned me about him. One was that he felt that he was still able to have sex which could end up infecting more people, and two, that he seemed to preach the gospel of gay too much. It was almost as if he was some spy or missionary who felt he could convert people to his choice of lifestyle. All the while, Jeff was trying to convince Don that if he prayed for him, he would stop being HIV positive and even stop being gay.

Jeff and I ended up having a lot of problems keeping that apartment. For some reason, the lock on our door broke, and someone was bold enough to not only come in and steal our cable descrambler, but also came right into my room while I was sleeping to take my watch. Part of my illness is that I have horrible nightmares (some stemming from never feeling safe as a child from physical abuse), and it became very hard for me to rest in that place. It wasn't the life I was used to, but in some ways, I was doing well there because I had people around and I was getting out, working, and helping Don with his business. Jeff would often do things that made the situation worse, though. For example, one night while half asleep, (as many people who take medications do), I woke up starving. I went to the fridge and saw some liver paste-one of my favorite foods-put it on some bread, and started to eat it. It turned out it was cat food Jeff had left in the fridge, and I nearly threw up when I realized it. It isn't a nice thing to say, but in a lot of ways Jeff was dumb as a sack of hammer handles. I suppose that doesn't say much for my own intelligence either mistaking cat food for liver paste. The long and short of it all was that I realized being around someone like that in the place you call home can be extremely stressful so I opted to get another apartment by myself. That was another mistake that nearly cost me everything, but I had the blinders on over my eyes. I missed being able to sleep all day, read all night and worry about only myself.

Soon I would have a new job, and a new place to live in and I tried to put all that garbage behind me. Sadly, some things just can't be put behind when a person is mentally ill. You must keep taking medication every single day, not drink alcohol at all, and take it very easy on yourself. These simple things can be hard to do, and hard to accept as permanent rules. I often wish I had broken down sooner and had found a group home where a healing and growing process could happen as it did later in life. I would have had so much more opportunities to do the things I wanted, like travel, save money, own a car. Maybe even have taken that Journalism course I had been so keen on as a youth. But the honest fact is, I went through a lot at that time, and for the rest of my days, it shaped who I am as a person.

Chapter Six: All Torn Up Inside

My next apartment was a third story place just a half a block from my church. I remember getting a lot out of the church services; I went to the adult Sunday school, studied my Bible, and volunteered for different things. Still, I was a bit of a rough character when compared to some of the people that went there. It seemed like they were always asking me odd questions, like did I go to the Persian Gulf War and why did I not have a decent paying job. It always seemed like people were either belittling me or trying to catch me in a lie. There was even a time some of the church people came over and went into my bathroom and went through the medications I take. In all the time, I went there I never felt accepted, and out of a congregation of some 1,200 people, I only made a small handful of lasting friendships.

While I had this new apartment, I started to discover the Internet, very slowly, because I had no one to teach me anything. I had put an ad in a local free ad newspaper asking for a second-hand IBM computer and printer, and someone called me with just what I was looking for, for just $100. I did a lot of typing on it, keeping a journal and writing my stories and printing them up. I also entered a lot of poetry contests but never won any of them. Everything about fiddling with computers was so exciting back then because it was such a quantum leap from pre-Internet days. Even just hooking up to something called the 'freenet' where you get monochrome access to things like chat rooms and text search engines was astonishing. At the time, I was writing poetry and reading a lot of it because I had figured that if I could write one page with a rhythmical and enlightening verse to it, I could adapt those abilities to writing a book. If I could do this, I thought, the book would end up to be a masterpiece of word-craftsmanship . The only problem was that while I was meeting more and more people online in chat rooms and on message boards, in the real world I was isolating myself more and more, and was finding it tough to discipline myself to write more than a few hours a week.

Soon after I got my new apartment, I decided I was getting well enough to go out and find a job. My doctor had put me on a new medication, a 'miracle' anti-depressant which helped me a lot. It had some funny qualities to it. I would wake up and take it in the morning and then go back to sleep, and I would have dreams that were all sunshine and rainbows, sugar and spice. Then I would get up and play video games or watch TV, or more likely, plug myself into the Internet. This process went on for a while, but when I decided I wanted more money and was fit and ready to try to work again, I got a job as a telephone sales person.

The work was stressful and taxing. I would sit in front of a computer screen, (just like at home) and the second I hung up on one call, the dialing software fed me another. You have to talk like crazy and be ready to come up with answers for any question a person could pose, always trying to sound calm and convincing. The money was good, well above the minimum wage, and there were bonuses to be made. I liked the people there, or at least most of them. I often had a chance to play jokes on customers, though some of them I probably shouldn't have done. One time a lady was very upset at me and became abusive, and instead of taking her off our list I sent her file to be called first after our next break. I could hear her screaming at the guy who answered the call, and he didn't find it funny, but I nearly pissed myself laughing. A lot of people find some of my pranks to be immature, but I have always felt that when things got stressful, a little laughter in a tough situation can help get you through. The whole time I worked there, I drank coffee after coffee, and I would work myself up into a state of mania (as in manic-depression or bipolar). The boss loved me, but I was playing dangerous games with my sanity. Some people wonder, considering my mental state, if I should have been working at all, but for me it was the choice between isolating myself and not having enough to eat and doing something that got me out of the house, got me meeting people and putting food on my table.

One time after work I had a few people come over to my bachelor pad and one of them showed me a few tricks and methods of improving my Internet experience. We all were having a lot of fun playing video games and swapping stories. This was the reason I got a difficult and menial job, to have these experiences again. One of the things I am kind of glad to have grown out of is that each time I meet a female I liked, I used to see her as a potential relationship. There was a young woman from work there that night and I let her know I was interested in her. Maybe it was because the relationship I had with Debbie a couple of short years before seemed to take me to such new levels of happiness and love that I desperately wanted to find that kind of commitment again.

The staff turnover in my new job was unreal. Sometimes we would be sitting and working, and people were getting fired who were sitting right next to us. Our boss had this theory that with the telemarketing computers that sent us calls the second it connected with a voice, we should have five times the bookings people used to make with manual dialing. Of course, he was wrong. The pressure of job loss and the need for constant performance is simply poison to just about anyone, more so for someone like me who suffers from a chronic mental illness.

I was only there for maybe a total of one month, and, among many others, two teenage girls, ages 17 and 18, were hired. One night they invited me to come with them to the bar, and the one who seemed to be interested in me, had her ex-boyfriend tag along with us. All the while they were arguing and I soon realized that there was a possibility the blonde liked me but wanted to make her ex-boyfriend jealous of me. Before the night ended, I bowed out and in a terrible late fall snowstorm I ended up walking halfway across the city in light clothes to get home.

Debbie was keeping in touch, she would even stop by now and then and I had a lot of strong feelings for her still. I often think she would have been the perfect match for me and that it had been my own ego that had kept us from going further than we did. I had such a hard time laying down any kind of commitment to her. I even went so far as to tell her about a woman from my past who once liked me that I had a very hard time not thinking about. It pains me now to think of hurting her. Debbie has been such a wonderful part of my life ever since the first day we met. I'm willing to accept that we may never have the relationship we once did just to keep our precious friendship going.

I knew I wasn't destined to be a telephone solicitor for the rest of my days and so I put in an application to a security guard service. I got a job with them in no time and worked a few shifts in hospitals, watching over patients who needed constant supervision. The security company sent me to a lot of different assignments at hospitals. One time I had to be a 'constant' for a guy who had a tube in his head called a shunt, and I had to remind him over and over not to play with it or try to pull it out. Another time I was working in Emergency watching a guy who was extremely belligerent who had fallen asleep outside after taking an overdose of pills and fell asleep on the wet ground for such a long time his butt was rotted. He kept claiming mistreatment and kept saying that I had better stop looking at him, and yelling about how painful his ass was. I'm very much ashamed of some of the things I have said and done in sheer ignorance of those who suffer from mental health issues. I don't know how I could have eased this person's pain, but a few choice words could have done a lot when I simply acted like a typical guard. I like to believe, I have grown since then. I also see the world's view of mentally ill people changing, and it means there is a lot of hope out there. In a way, I was proud to work in situations like this, and most of the time I would end up being friends with the people I guarded. It didn't help, though, when I had to turn around and try and get admitted as a psychiatric patient to places where I once worked.

One guy wasn't in the hospital for any Psychiatric purpose, but for whatever reason, he was just angry with everyone and had a bad attitude about everything. At one point I was asked to steady his arm so an IV line could be put in and while I was holding his arm he spat in my face. The worst of all of them, though, was guarding a young kid who was stabbed seven times, five of them in his back. He was not more than 17 and must have been going through hell. I was guarding him because he had some serious troubles with the law. In the morning a prosecutor was going to come down and lay charges on him. Poor kid was so young and had badly messed up his whole life, not to mention that he was very close to having been murdered. I remember looking at him and thinking that he was still lucky to be alive and said a few prayers for him silently.

There were easy ones, too. I loved that I could sit and sometimes read a whole book in just a night or two. I ran through novels like water, reading some great spy stuff and different parts of the Bible. I also loved legal dramas and historical works. I got a decent education from sitting around in those hospital wards.

After a few months, the security guard company must have figured me as being trustworthy, because I was given two regular 12-hour shifts on the weekend at a Steel Mill on the South Side of the City. The only thing wrong was that I lived on the North Side of the city, and it sometimes took two hours each way to get to and from work. The first shift was okay, but halfway through the second shift, I would be pretty exhausted. I did have a kind supervisor, though. She was an older lady, very close to retirement who had leukemia and didn't expect to even see her first day of retirement one or two years down the road.

The job seemed pretty good, but there was a lot of walking involved, and I was still using my cane, which didn't help much. Nothing helped my knees except resting them most of the time. Then I would have to exercise them as much as I could until they got sore again. Working in that mill was murder on them. They would crack and pop and feel like they were falling apart. Still, I soldiered on.

After being there a while, lights from a car would shine across the parking lot in front of where I sat at some point in my shift . Then sometimes a light on the switchboard would indicate a phone in use somewhere in the plant. After a couple of months of wondering if I was paranoid or not, one of the field supervisors, who drives around in the security cars responding to alarms and checking up on people, came in and asked for my paperwork. I gave it to him, and then I told him about what had been happening. He said that because I talked about computers and sometimes brought a small computer to work with me, one of my fellow employees had told the security office that I was hacking into the computers in the office of the steel mill, and printing up paycheques. Nothing could have been more ridiculous. The computer I had was in no way even close to being compatible with the ones in the office, and I would never even attempt such a thing at that time because I had such limited, self-taught knowledge of computing. The idea that they would spy on me and try to charge me with something seemed so freaking ridiculous.

My life at that time was getting to be harder and more stressful for me. My parents had moved to a small town 30 km further away than the small city I grew up in, and sometimes I would have to beg my dad to give me a ride home so I could get home soon enough to sleep eight hours before my next shift. The stress of having to stay awake all night wired on coffee and spied on by supervisors, despite being completely alone, was intense. My dad and I were fighting a lot, which hurt because we had been such a close family before my illness manifested itself and drove a wedge between me and anyone who cared about me. I was trying to seek some self-respect by working, and my dad was having a very hard time making ends meet for him and my mom. Sometimes the arguments we had would involve shouting, and my dad would get so angry he would kick me out of his car. More than once, I had to walk home from the middle of downtown-far from any bus route or the warm comfort of my apartment. I feel so thankful that I have grown as a person enough to have a job that fulfills me and doesn't ask the impossible.

I can remember being so stressed out and so homesick for coastal living that one day I just packed up and went to the airport and tried to get a flight to Vancouver. I couldn't afford a ticket to the coast, but I did get a ticket to Calgary, a sister city to Edmonton about three hours' drive south of where I lived. I got there and tried to look up a cousin who used to live there, but he had gone to some other far off place, and when I decided I wouldn't find him I took a bus to the mountains and stayed in a traveler's Hostel in the incredibly beautiful city of Banff. It felt so good to be going somewhere, to be seeing new things and getting out of the grind of work. But of course the work, no matter how hard it was-isolating, depressing, mind-numbing-it paid for that trip.

I think it was within a short while of that trip that I had made the decision that I didn't need my anti-depressant medications anymore. Taking yourself off medication is common but almost never works in the patient's favor. What often happens is the drug works and works well, and then you think you are better and don't need it anymore. It was a grave mistake, and I quickly started slipping mentally. Working those two 12-hour shifts completely isolated wasn't helping. I was also having a hard time making it to church or youth service. My job was putting food on my table, and video games in my living room, but it was giving me one sure-fire recipe for disaster: isolation, loneliness and severe stress added to a disrupted sleep schedule. I became extremely depressed over time, and there was nothing to lift me out of it. I did have one friend, a guy named Mike who was considerably older but very sharp minded and kind. He was a gun collector and had me over and showed me some cool weapons: everything from a WWII German Luger to a shotgun used by modern day U.S. Marines that had a laser sight on it. He was a very helpful guy and wanted to get me a more modern computer, something I felt I would do just about anything to get. Anything but what happened to Mike.

One day I had a knock at the door, and I didn't want to answer it because I hadn't let anyone in the building. I looked through the viewer and saw that it was two middle aged guys in suits. I opened the door, and they said they were Homicide Detectives and they almost immediately started asking me questions about Mike. I asked them to stop and then asked them if someone had murdered Mike. They looked at each other with surprise and then told me he was dead.

I invited them in, answered their questions and printed up my Journals so they could see what I had been doing over the past few days. One of them, the 'bad cop' of the two, assured me that they would be back and that I should cancel any plans I may have had to leave town. It felt a little grim, but it seemed obvious that the cop thought I was my friend's murderer.

Eventually, even the problem with the Police blew over. A while after that, as I became more and more depressed, I picked up the phone book and looked up the young woman I had met at a summer camp as a teen. I hadn't seen her in person in years, and we hadn't talked in a long time. I hoped and prayed she could forgive me; that time did heal all wounds. I wanted to tell her about the summer camp I was a counselor at, about how things had changed in the years since she dropped me as a friend, that my medication was working and that I would never be sick again, no matter how big of a lie that was. I also wanted desperately to say that I needed her. I called, and she answered, and I said my name and the line went silent. I said,

"Well, you haven't screamed and hung up yet, that's good news." My heart sunk. I knew she had no intention of letting me back into her life.

We talked for a while, but at the end of the conversation, she implied that she had no interest in talking to me further and that she considered me to be a psychopath. That was a knife in the chest. I hung up the phone devastated, feeling desperately alone and depressed. Over time, the idea that I had no romantic hope in this world started to get to me. I had lost Debbie and now this girl that had meant so much to me. Add to that the effect of the withdrawal of my antidepressant medication, and I decided I was going to kill myself. I didn't want to do it as a cry for help, but as an act of someone with no hope left. If I had stayed on my antidepressants there would have been no question of such a conclusion for me. I took almost a full bottle of Acetaminophen and some other drugs from my medicine cabinet. As I got more sedated from the effect of the drugs, I took more. When I started to feel tired, I put a plastic bag over my head and lay down in bed thinking I could suffocate myself. The bag didn't do its job, so I managed to keep breathing, but I slept for two days. When I woke up, I felt like I had been knocked cold by a blunt force trauma and threw up many times. Then I went back to sleep and woke up a day later. I heard someone knocking at the door, and ignored it and let them leave then went to the bathroom and noticed they had slipped a $20 bill under my door.

For the next while, I could hold nothing down, not even a sip of water. I didn't think I was going to die but knew if it was to happen, that this would be an awful way to do it, so I called up the poison control hotline and told them what had happened. They told me I was very likely in serious trouble and that I had better get to the hospital. If it hadn't been for my dad putting that money for cab fare under my door, I don't know what might have happened. I was taken to the hospital and put in intensive care where I spent the next few days. My doctor had told my family that I would be dead in a short while. My sister even called from Toronto and talked about coming to visit me. This offer was a surprise because I had not been welcome in my sister's home since my very first breakdown many years before that. It is very hard to find meaning to such a desperate act, but one thing I have to say is that while lying in that hospital bed I saw how much my family really did care. Not long after, my brother told me that he saw me as a Christ figure, though Jesus didn't try to take his own life and my brother and I knew and understood I wasn't anyone divine. It was just something that he felt as he saw me nearly die and how it brought everyone to understand how much we needed each other.

The next few days were touch and go. No one had told me I was dying, but I knew I was very sick. It hurt so much to see my mom standing by my side crying her eyes out and my brother and dad being so nice to me. Somehow I meditated and prayed, and for whatever reason, I defied what the doctor had said and walked home to my apartment two days later. I did have stomach pains for a while, but mostly I was healthy. I don't know why, but they didn't transfer me to a Psychiatric Ward after that. Sometimes, I think of the theory in Physics and Philosophy about choices. In this theory, each time we reach a fork in the road destiny creates two Universes. In one of them we take a left, and in the other, we take a right, and this effect goes on and on in billions of alternate Universes-every choice or movement we make. As I write this now, I sometimes wonder about dying in that hospital bed and the chance that the life I have now is Purgatory. I suppose if it were,

I would never really know. All I do know is that I would never put my family through that pain again, it seems such a selfish thing to take your life. Everyone suffers but you.

Three last events from that part of my life stand out. One was finding a newspaper article that stated that Don had been acquitted. Don was the gay guy who lived upstairs from me when I lived with Jeff. His charge was knowingly infecting a former lover with HIV. The second event was being a witness at the murder trial of my friend Mike. The last happened after I got out of the hospital. My dad gave me his old car, and it played a big role in becoming close friends with Debbie again. Another leg of my journey was about to begin, where I would form new and better relationships with both Debbie, my brother, my sister, and parents.

Chapter Seven: My Closest Companion

Not long after I got my Dad's old car up and running, I got a new job with an outfit that had been doing security since the days of cowboys and masked bandits. When I went into the office to apply, I noticed the Operations Manager had a bunch of pictures up from his former army unit. He turned out to be a fascinating guy, and we talked for half an hour or more about the military, and I left feeling as though I had made a friend. I must have because he called me the very next day to hire me. He liked to add a sense of adventure to the work, often calling me up and saying, "Your assignment, should you choose to accept it..." He ended up being one of the best bosses I ever had. I hate to say it, but if it hadn't been for him, I would have never lasted in the job. He knew early on that I had a mental illness and did me many favors, covering my screw-ups and giving me as little or as much work as I could handle.

My first job with that company was to sit in my car and keep an eye on a trucking company. As I sat there, negotiations for the sale of the company were going on. My boss gave me one of the old 'brick' cell phones and the phone number of the vice president of the company that was buying the trucking company. The concern was that they were going to sell the place and sneak all the more valuable stuff out the back door rather than include it all in the sale price. It is rare that a security job gets interesting, and while this one showed promise, it ended up being a long, boring assignment.

It took a lot out of me to sit in my car for 12 hours a day, always staying alert. I wasn't getting paid a lot, but I had respect for what I was doing, which is much better than sitting at home watching your life roll by, playing video games or going into chat rooms on a computer. One thing that made a huge difference in this job was that I was guaranteed to get a surprise visit from one of the mobile supervisors on every shift. It gave me a reason to stay on my toes. Still, though, I was on heavy medications and experiencing depression and stress to the extreme. Each day I would work those long hours, then come home to an empty apartment. I wonder if I caused myself to be alone because I was depressed. I do remember going through stages of isolating myself to in some way punish myself when I was depressed. Sometimes I also got it in my head that if I went drinking, I would solve my problems. It took me years to learn my lesson, but I eventually found out that mixing alcohol with medications is never a solution. It was just that I had so many good memories from my teen years of going out, loosening up with a few drinks and being able to connect with my friends and ask girls to dance who I would never have normally had the courage to approach. On medications, even a couple of drinks would leave me sick for days.

I worked at the trucking company, trying to spend as much time as I could with Debbie until my car's engine seized up and I was unable to pay to fix it. Then I went back to working as a stationary guard. A lot of my assignments after that focused on two high-rise condo apartment buildings, which were excellent places to work. One of them was a posh condo complex that a friend from my hometown lived in, and the other had a lot of people who were friendly and down to earth. I got to know many of them. In the second building was another friend from school and when he would go out on a Friday night, he would always say he was going to meet his future ex-wife. He often joked that he would buy me a hooker if I let him throw loud parties, although I was never really sure he was joking.

At the time, I was still very naïve. I had a pretty screwed up idea of how to ask out women or let them know I liked them. There was a group of people who once approached me because they came home one day and I was at my desk, in uniform, sitting in the lobby of the building, reading my Bible. I didn't want to change churches at that point, but one of the women in the group made some indications of liking me, and I wanted to try and get to know her better. I came up with some foolish ideas, like buying her a necklace and giving it to her anonymously. I might have tried some of these lame ideas, but as a security guard and I like to think a gentleman. I had always respected the privacy of others. This attitude was crucial, especially with the job I had.

That year, and for a while until just a few years ago, my thoughts seemed to be stuck on a young woman I had known in adolescence. We weren't even acquaintances, though she was kind to me on numerous occasions. I wish I knew what type of mental illness this kind of obsession is because I would gladly take pills for it. It isn't just something that happened to me either, I have known quite a few people with severe mental illnesses of many different types who are 'stuck' on a concept of a person (almost never the person themselves.) My delusional relationship nearly caused me some serious problems, especially because of my loneliness. I had written to her a few times, but she had never written back. I had even run into her a few times but didn't say anything. Around Christmas, I tried to write her another letter and sent it off and seriously thought the police were going to arrest me because of it. I even called up the police to turn myself in. They didn't come for me, but I did get word that her father had said I was harassing her. My mind made up all kinds of excuses to try and justify this harsh reaction, hoping that they hadn't labeled me as some horrible person who harassed innocent young women. I didn't write any more letters for a long time, not until when I was sick again, and all my old delusions came back. Strangely, I was actively pursuing other women who often responded well to me, and the young woman I wrote to hadn't shown any interest in me other than some flirting in a bar some ten years before. Still, my troubled mind led me to believe that she cared in some way for me. I think if one were to try and analyze it, her flirtations in that bar came at a time when I was susceptible to just about any kind of unusual treatment and the surprise of a woman like this showing desire for me imprinted a false reality deep into my subconscious mind.

Soon after this letter writing incident, a friend of mine from church who was single bought a huge house and invited me to be his roommate. He hadn't picked the liveliest part of town to get a house in, but I thought I would enjoy living there more than my current place, so I moved in. The place was massive. It had a patio upstairs and another downstairs, it had five bedrooms and three bathrooms, two huge living rooms, and on and on. It was a bit of a bonus that the friend who owned the place was a great guy and he had a degree in

Psychology, which I thought would be of benefit if I needed someone to talk to abut my problems.

Up until then I had some pretty small places and thought these cramped, noisy or dirty apartments were contributing to my depression, but often I would find myself pacing around this big new house until my knees were hurting, trying to clear my head or deal with some of my black moods. I remember in one of my first apartments going to the laundry room and sitting in the dark while I was deep down in the dumps. I thought somehow that if I just had a different place things would be better. The simple fact was that it was hard to get a proper mix of medication that kept away my paranoia and depression and dealt with my mood swings. There was another factor, that although I had wanted to, I was unable to find a real psychologist or counsellor to talk to about my problems and help me manage my life. No matter how beautiful or large or filled with money or food or beer, it wasn't going to do anything for my mental health.

As mentioned, my roommate Steve was a good friend and a caring person. He did have enough money to buy that huge house but was far from rich. Steve had gotten a three-year psychology degree and then started his own landscaping business. He had come from a farm in Northern British Columbia, and he was the hardest working person I have ever met. One time he and I went to cut down a tree for one of his clients, and I stayed on the ground while he climbed about 25 feet up a tree with a chainsaw tied to his waist, cutting branches as he went. I wouldn't even attempt it with full climbing gear. He thought nothing of it.

It did eventually get unbearable to live in that house. Steve was always coming up with new rule sheets saying I had to sit down to pee and organize my stuff the way he wanted, and all kinds of such things. I spent a lot of time watching TV, working on my computer, drinking coffee, and occasionally going out for a cigarette, but there were times when I could have used a sympathetic ear. Most of the time, though, my roommate would be downstairs watching his TV if hockey was on or playing hockey video games on his game console. Talking to him was like talking to a brick wall. I only have myself to blame, but I felt really stressed out not having anything to do, any work or anyone to talk to and so I turned to the bottle a couple of times to try and jump start my moods. I can remember still being in the whole mindset of having to go to a party or a dance club on the weekends and I wasted time, money, and brain cells finding out that was no help either. I just couldn't seem to shake the idea that finding a relationship with a woman would be the solution to all of my problems. There was another thing that I think played a part and that was being addicted to excitement, adrenalin.

One of the things I did that perhaps wasn't so bad was that I bought a powerful CO_2 pellet pistol and would practice with it in the garage. At that time, I still hadn't gotten over my obsession with the military and could do that sort of thing for hours at a time. Steve also kept alcohol in the house, but just fruity-type juice coolers.

Another thing I would sometimes do that was likely just as harmful if not more so, was play video lottery terminals. Just a couple of years before that I wouldn't think of gambling, but then I started visiting Debbie's sister who worked at a restaurant that had these evil machines, and we would often play them together when she got off work. For a while, there seemed to be no harm in it, for the first while it seemed I won more than I lost. There was also one time I was lined up to play and one of the people ahead of me was the former mayor of my hometown.

It was incredible how those machines would get to a person. You fire in dollar coin after dollar coin, the lights go off, the stereo speakers click out the sound of each win or loss of a quarter. When I played them I often felt an incredible rush of energy. Then I started to lose a lot and managed to quit until I moved into Steve's house.

All the while as these things were going on, I had been searching for easy ways to get rich. One time I ran across some information about a company that sold and serviced 1-900 numbers. There were numbers for weather and numbers for sports picks, everyone thought that 1-900 numbers were the wave of the future (since the Internet had not yet taken off). I had even heard of a guy who owned one number and set it to charge the maximum amount. He would then go around asking to borrow phones at a business or residence, and make his living calling his own number. Some of these bills would run into the hundreds of dollars. There just seemed to be no honest way I could make enough to live on and have a decent life, other than working myself to death.

Hoping I could somehow shoestring my way into the 1-900 number market, I took all my electronics to a local pawn shop, borrowed a few hundred with it, then bought a money order and sent it off to a 1-900 company. After a while, I realized this would be nearly impossible to market and advertise, and it would also be hard dealing with the stress of it all, and I was going through quite a bit of that already. I could handle my part-time security job. Stress when working was manageable, and my boss would give me time off if needed. Running a business was something entirely different. I ended up canceling the order to the 1-900 company and still came up too short of money to redeem my possessions from the pawn shop.

I was undaunted in my quest for the easy millions. I was hoping that somehow I could make a better life for myself despite my psychiatric disability. I kept reading the papers and found an ad for a marketing college that sounded good. I phoned them and made an appointment and went down and they gave me a test which was so simple a border collie could pass it, and I took home a student loan application. School started, and since a friend had once come to me to be partners in a business venture, when the instructor asked us to introduce ourselves, I announced that I was a senior partner of Phoenix Forest Products. It was true, but it wasn't a million dollar a day company. It was an idea-my friend never even registered it as a business and he printed up some cards for it on his home computer. A couple of days later my student loan was refused because I still hadn't paid back my loan from flying school when I had lived in BC. The other problem was that the school wanted us all to dress in business attire, and though my parents were good enough to buy me one set of dressy clothes, I was ashamed that I would have had to come dressed like that every day, so the easiest thing became dropping out.

This type of reaction is an example of how mental health stigma affects those who have a disorder. Everyone wants to hide their illness; it leads to discrimination in the workplace, lost opportunities and many other negative consequences. I was so concerned that others would know I was mentally ill and living on a disability income that I invented lies, and half-truths. I wanted to make it look like I was a wealthy business person and had a lot of money. I wanted to make everyone think that I was as far from being mentally ill as anyone could be. But when it came down to it, I didn't even have clothes for school and the whole house of cards folded. Fortunately, in this situation, it was likely a good thing that I dropped out because I was told later by a friend that the school was putting on a scam and there were a lot of lies the school had told their students. I just wish I could have completed something, seen something through. I had dropped out of school, I had unfinished correspondence courses lying around, and a string of jobs I had lost because I couldn't fulfill my commitments. Somehow, at some point I just stopped caring about keeping my word and trying to be responsible. I felt as though the harsh treatment I had received in psychiatric hospitals and wards showed that society had betrayed me first, while in fact I had an illness and they had done everything in their power to make me better.

Soon after that, I got sick of living in that vast empty house I was in and found an apartment that was a massive 900 square feet and very close to not only the church I attended at the time, but a few friends, including Dunzel. From that point on it seemed my gambling problem kept getting worse. I even sat down and taught myself one of the simpler computer languages so I could run simulations on beating roulette. I spent a lot of time behind the computer in that apartment, a good deal of it writing the book that came before this one. Though I did benefit from the new location, I would soon learn that such changes don't always result in me getting the things I needed. I think likely at that time what I needed was an anti-depressant that worked and a group of friends. I remember when I wasn't at the computer I would sit in my comfortable chair eating snacks and playing cassettes and CDs from my growing music collection. Little did I know that one day when I had been through some wringers, my life would improve to a point I could almost never imagine. I was to have a pretty tough next few years, though.

Chapter Eight: Big Scary Dude

One night when I was in my new two-bedroom apartment, a young woman who was a friend of Dunzel's came by late at night. She was endearing, fun, and easy to get along with, though I suspect treatment for depression would have helped her a lot. I had met her before. Dunzel had a crush on her for some time, but for whatever reason, she kept going back to an old boyfriend who was a total creep. His name was Bill, and the first time I had met him he was laying on Dunzel's floor, and he asked me if I had any downers on me. When I said no he tried to sell me his leather jacket which I think he had found in a garbage somewhere. Liz, his girlfriend, went through so much shit for him it was unreal. At one point, they went to Jasper together, a small mountain community 350 km west of Edmonton, and he ended up getting jail time for assaulting her. Still, she kept seeing him.

It is a funny thing: the ego of a man. I suppose this happens to a lot of men but sometimes a guy will pick out a woman to pursue, and they count that potential as a sure thing. With Liz, I figured if I were as nice and as stable a guy as possible, and was her true friend, that one day I would have her as my girlfriend. I once knew a person who used to talk to women as though they had already agreed to marry him, saying things like, "That's just what I need is a woman who knows how to handle money." I'm not sure if it was the way he talked, his looks or his personality, but he got more women than I ever did.

In the case of Liz, I was very interested, and somehow we did seem to click. I was even further impressed because Dunzel had gotten her a modeling job where she was earning $500 an hour plus free clothes. Still, she never seemed happy. One night she called me up and asked me to come over, and while I was there we chatted a bit, then she went into the other room for a while, and then she came back and said, "Leif, I am such a baby. Do you think you could come and sleep with me?"

It seemed a simple enough thing. Most people don't have any problem sleeping with a $500 an hour fashion model. I told her that I had to go back to my apartment to get my medications, and she came along, and we laid down and I held her close. We kissed a little, but she stopped me, and I was happy enough just to lay next to her, so I didn't try to push my luck and held her until she fell asleep. It was kind of a beautiful thing to experience, but it left me with a lot of unanswered questions: a confused view of my relationship with her, and feelings of not being sure about my place in the world. Maybe I was getting older and didn't have the looks I used to count on. Maybe it was like she said and she just wasn't attracted to men with short hair. Who knows?

I got up and went back to my favorite chair and sat quietly listening to music until it was time to wake her and drive her home. I let her off and then headed for the highway and kept going. I drove so far I ended up in a small town I had never been to before and checked into a hotel. It was kind of a pleasant experience to be able to get away and get my head together. I told a doctor a lie about needing one day's worth of medications, and he gave me a prescription. On the way out I stopped to ask his secretary if there was a swimming pool in town. She got up, came and sat down next to me, looked me in the eyes and touched my knee as she told me the directions. She was a pretty nice looking woman who helped give my confidence a boost. I kind of needed one after Liz pushed me away the night before. As time has gone by, I don't need to be constantly complimented or get signals that females are interested in me. I don't know why it was so important to me in my early 20s other than that I had a fear of ending up alone. I did end up alone, I think mostly because I was beset by mental illness at such a crucial age. I was barely past adolescence and hadn't learned anything about forming strong relationships, I didn't even have many friends to speak of, and becoming severely ill stunted my social development.

It was so relaxing to get that hotel room, a little cell with a TV and a bathtub. I took a long, relaxing, hot bath, enjoying the soft water and laid around eating popcorn. All the while I was thinking, "If I could spend a month in this little cave I would." Not tell anyone I was gone but my parents, just live anonymously for a little while. I often think that if I ever get another credit card and the means to pay it off, I would take off on long trips like that all the time. For many years, I have actively wanted to discover the highways and cities and towns of the US like in Jack Kerouac novels or one of my favorite books ever, "Travels with Charley," the Nobel Prize-winning book by John Steinbeck.

I got back to Edmonton the next day, and all was as normal. I felt better, and more able to handle the fact that I had pursued someone who I cared for and didn't send her off screaming in the other direction. I loved living in a large apartment, but after time I would go to doing things only the loneliest people do-like going through phone books looking for people to talk to from my past. One of the people I called was an old Cadet friend named Peter who was at the time living in a Military Base East of Edmonton and flying one of the world's most advanced fighter jets. We talked for a long time about our time in Cadets, and he even spoke to me about some of the planes Canada has. The neat thing about him telling me this was that I had pictures of most of those planes posted around my kitchen where I liked to sit and play my music and smoke.

Peter was quite a nice guy. I didn't think he would have wanted to associate with me, but at the end of our conversation, he told me that he had a house on the base and plenty of extra room if I ever wanted to stay over. I wanted to just preserve that offer in some non-decaying agent, so I never took him up on it. I was so worried that if I let him know I was a psychiatric patient, it would ruin what little friendship we had from the past and over the phone. I called him a few times after that. I even asked him half-jokingly if he could take me up in an F-18. He said if I were still in the military I could take a course called "high-altitude indoctrination," and he could get me a ride. I would have liked to have been able to do that. Ever since my flying days, I dreamed of one day flying a powerful fighter jet or even getting a ride in one. I was amazed to learn later that the F-18 produces somewhere around 1/3 the thrust of the space shuttle. One time I had watched one at an air show fly slowly past the crowd at not even a hundred feet, and then hit the engines and afterburners all at once and blast off so high, it couldn't be seen, all to the tune of the Kenny Loggins song, "Danger Zone." Sadly, I never did get that chance at my dream ride. The amazing thing, though, is that if a person keeps trying, goes on battling their demons-mine being a mental illness-new dreams come and sometimes become reality. I laugh now when I look back to the time I thought random typing on a keyboard was sending messages to the radio station because modern computers and the Internet have made such things such a small part of computing just about anyone understands it as possible. Flying was a fun adventure for a while, but I think I was destined for bigger things, like writing and publishing my books and giving mental health talks to large audiences, all the while having the friends and co-workers I could only have dreamed of having a short time before. All that gives a sense of satisfaction that I don't think any supersonic plane could ever give me.

After living in that apartment for some time, I got to meet my neighbor across the hall. He was a man in his 40s, tall with dark hair and a mustache, and he was just about the worst person I had ever met in my life. He seemed okay at first. He kept a clean house. He even gave me a spare key to his apartment in case he got locked out, and he offered me the use of his bike. One time I took him to the graveyard to see his father's grave and I felt a kind of special friendship with him after that.

Then one day he knocked on my door and came in and told me he was high on cocaine. He had some pot on him and offered me some, but I wasn't interested. He left and then a few minutes later phoned me and asked me to come over. I went to his place, and my jaw dropped when this 6'4" former debt collector was wearing nothing but a housecoat and watching gay porn. I am almost too ashamed to remember it, but he started to come on to me and even tried to force me to stay in his apartment. I left, then he called again and said he was sorry, and asked me to come and see him. I stupidly did, and he made another play for me.

I went back to my apartment and the phone wouldn't stop ringing. I didn't answer it but checked the voicemail messages, and on the voice recording, he kept saying things like, "Please Leif, let me suck your dick. I promise it won't hurt. I'll be gentle. If you don't do it, I'll say bad things about you. Come on, I'm on more anti-depressants than you are." I got disgusted to the point of nausea and called the police. They came down, and he called right while they were there. Thankfully they arrested him, but I was too embarrassed to appear as a witness. I took solace in the fact that the cops downloaded and saved the messages and likely had a good time passing around a tape of him at the cop shop. For a long time, I felt very violated from all of this. I was still in the mindset then that there is no such thing as people who are entirely bad. I should have likely seen this guy for what he was when I first met him from the things he told me about being a debt collector and a drug and alcohol abuser. Not only was I extremely troubled by this near sexual assault, but I longed to go back to my hometown of St. Albert where it seemed that things like this never happened.

After having the police arrest him, I talked to the owner of the building who had the ability to evict someone with 24 hours' notice if they posed a danger to other tenants. He said that there was nothing he would do except evict me because I was behind on my rent at the time. I moved, which is likely what the landlord wanted. I got a smaller but much more affordable apartment in another part of town with seemingly friendly and sociable caretakers and settled into living in a much better area in a much nicer building. It didn't hurt that there was a pool hall and a discount bookstore just down the street.

Summer came soon, and I spent a lot of time working on my writing and discovering the new world of the Internet.

Chapter Nine: Self Torture Plus Shame

The place I moved to was nicely kept up. The paint was fresh, the carpet was clean and comfortable, and I managed to bring over enough furniture to meet all my needs. The only problem was that I was desperately lonely. Within a short while, I started going to the pool hall a lot and nursing a coffee which eventually led to drinking beer again. It never seemed to strike me that if I didn't go to a bar or other place where drinking and gambling went on, I likely wouldn't have these slips. Five years ago I had my last taste of beer and decided it was time to get serious. For a year I went to meetings almost every day and wouldn't allow myself to go in bars or think about alcohol. It wasn't easy, but the mental and spiritual growth I experiences was worth every minute I spent in those meetings. The pool hall was a problem, and I shouldn't have gone there, but there were another couple of bars just within a block of there, and two of them had Video Lottery Terminals. For me, these were like what crystal meth is to an addict. When you are addicted to video lottery terminals and other forms of gambling, you can't stop thinking about loading these machines up and spinning the lucky reels. You also tend to keep thinking about when and where you will get your next money to play. The depths of sadness and guilt that comes about when you lose time and again without learning your lesson is frightening.

The worst time for me was when I had a little cash, and restlessness, boredom or loneliness started to set into my head. Some people say to watch out for when you are hungry, angry, lonely or tired. I had a craving for excitement, and these machines knew how to push my buttons. They were modern versions of one-armed bandits, more advanced, more computerized and sneaky. I would scrape together ten bucks, even pawn something to play; then I would go there and gamble right to my last quarter. What gets to me now is that I played these things for years, putting thousands into them in the intervals of insanity I experienced. In all this time, I had never hit the jackpot, the famous five sevens in a row. One day when I finally did get them, I suddenly realized that after all that, hitting the highest payout they have, my winnings were less than what I earned in a day as a stage hand. It was shortly after that I was finally able to put gambling behind me for good.

So many days went by when I was in a terrible state, where I would be so depressed and mad at myself for gambling my last money away. When these horrible feelings surfaced, I would sit in the small space of tile by my apartment door, head in hands, hating myself for being such a sick person. It was time to get help, and I ended up going to gambling abstinence meetings and seeing a counselor. It worked for a while, but often a few months down the road my resolve would melt again. Like with medication, I would decide I was no longer sick, or even just not care, and I would bet a $20 on the VLT machine, then start to chase my losses and take out all the money in my account and get a cab to the casino. A few times I came out ahead; many times I didn't.

In one of my periods of not gambling, a friend I met in a recovery class who seemed to be doing well for himself convinced me to go into a program at the Salvation Army for addictions. When looking back now, I think about how young I was, and how I liked to talk about how horrible my addiction was. People would often feel I needed more help than I let on, or at least it seemed that way. Nevertheless, I made the decision that I was going to go through with the program, and I went there with my friend. They accepted me and put me in a dorm room, and after taking my night medications, I tried to sleep. The problem was that half the guys in there were snoring, and I didn't like the idea of being exposed to some of the hardest of the hardcore addicts those kinds of places treat. The very next morning I checked myself out. The sad reality for me was that I was an addicted gambler, but also a person with a mental illness. I thought by solving the gambling problem I would be able to have all the things other people had that had gone through treatment, like a job and a future. Deep down internally, addiction or not, counseling program or not, I was still afflicted with both bipolar and schizoaffective disorder to the point where none of those goals were realistic. I was a messed up individual and the journey I had to follow would take everything I had because I needed to help myself out of the holes that nature and bad decisions had dug for me.

A while after that as I struggled with my addictions and loneliness, the Homicide Detectives from the Edmonton Police came to see me again. They told me they wanted to take me downtown to question me and so I went with them and was grilled for two hours. The cops didn't even say that they were videotaping me with a hidden camera. I tried to be as totally honest as I could. I even admitted to minor things I had done just to not look like a liar or that I was hiding something. I felt bad that Mike had been murdered. He was a very kind and intelligent guy and had some interesting hobbies, like playing chess and operating his computer bulletin board. Somehow, though, I felt numb to all this. My priority at the time was convincing these two guys that I wasn't a murderer.

While the gambling and the police business were going on, I was working for Pinkerton's in some more interesting assignments. I often worked at the Art Gallery and was exposed to a lot of interesting people and culture. Sometimes people from Europe would come there and insult us for having such a small and dull Art Gallery compared to the ones in London and Paris. One time, we had an open-door day on New Year's Eve, and a couple of police came in, and for some reason one of them walked up to a piece of art that was made of Plexiglas and knocked on it like he owned it. I went up to him and said, "Sir, can I please ask you not to touch the art?" I had to keep myself from snickering at the idea of me, this skinny kid who had been tossed around more than a few times by oversize police officers on my way to a psychiatric hospital, telling a cop what he could and couldn't do. He seemed to be put out by what I said, and tried to make a 'tough guy' comment, but couldn't say much and ended up leaving.

One time I worked outside at a car lot tent sale for seven straight days, 12 hours a day. It was perhaps the most I had ever worked. At the end of it, I went out and bought a gold-plated watch for myself with the money. A few days later I found the same watch for quite a bit less and went to the original store to get a refund and buy the cheaper one. They ended up just giving me about $80 which I promptly blew on another VLT binge. Things were getting worse, and I had no idea how to stop the problem. I just went to more meetings, and each time I gambled I tried to work enough to afford to eat and pay my rent. Putting myself through all this extra work and barely having enough to live was like I was torturing myself. I felt so much guilt and pain after I gambled. The losing and the psychological and financial trap I was in were at least as bad as my mental illness. I don't understand why I was so unable to stop, the rewards of fun and money weren't there at all. There is a theory that compulsive gamblers secretly want to punish themselves, which could be true.

.

One of the worst things about working as a security guard is that anyone who works where you do thinks they are your boss. As well, a lot of people react with anger and belligerence when someone in authority, especially in uniform is around. There was this one guy at a high-rise I was working at who came up to me saying that I had to put away my desk after every shift I worked because he wanted it that way and he was on the condo board. I got so frustrated at the idea of having to move furniture at his bidding that I ended up requesting a different place to work. Before I left, though, a guy who lived in the building, gave me a party invitation. I didn't end up going. I was sad to leave that building; I had made many friends there. I heard later that some of the young women who lived there were talking about me in the elevator, and there was one of them who I would have taken out if I had the chance. Sometimes, though, I wonder if being in a relationship would have solved anything. What I do know is that there were times after that when I became severely mentally ill. Would any of the women I connected with have had the compassion to see me through those times? Just thinking about how superficial I was, I think I would just have attracted another superficial person who never would have stuck by my side. These days, I often shun chances to connect with members of the opposite sex. I do this knowing they might not accept my peculiarities as a person with bipolar disorder and symptoms of schizophrenia. Also, I have done things that way because if I did get into a relationship and it had to end one day while I was sick, the devastation it would wreak on my psyche would be unbearable.

Those were sometimes happy days and sometimes crazy ones. Once I was sent to a yard owned by an oil company, and I was given use of a $50,000 flat-deck truck, and it had the sweetest radio. I listened to music, and talk shows all night and their regular patrol guard came by and we spoke for a while. He told me that there was a spaceship behind the Hale-Bopp comet that everyone could see with the naked eye and it was going to 'rescue' chosen people. I put my faith in him as much as I did the people who were trying to drum up fear that the end of the Mayan Calendar meant the world would end. It all came from a popular talk show host; he could be very convincing if you read a lot of science fiction.

After two years of service with Pinkerton's, I lost my job by not being able to show up for an assigned shift, and didn't have one for a while. The advantage of being a security guard is that there are so many come and go, fly by night outfits that if you want a break, a change, get fired or quit, there is always another company willing to hire you. I was sad to leave Pinkerton's; it was a well-organized and well-disciplined outfit. My bosses had always been good to me, and the supervisors all had some serious military experience. I think it was a good time for me to take a much-deserved rest from the pressures of night work.

Not long after my employment ended, a guy was moving into my building, and I jumped in and started helping him without asking for anything. I can't remember now, but I either got $20 or some free pizza and my new neighbor's eternal gratitude. He ran a gas station owned by his brother up the street from our building and one day in the pool hall he offered me a job. It seemed like it was the chance of a lifetime. I was extremely down those days, and the next day I was sitting by my radio, rolling and smoking cigarettes. My dad came by and saw me in my chair, hunched over, in a total funk, and he decided he was going to take me to the hospital right then and there. He called up my new boss and truthfully told him it broke my heart that I wasn't going to be able to work for him, and I ended up checking into the psychiatric ward to be treated for severe depression at the University Hospital. I was twenty-five at the time, and it seemed that my spirits rose as soon as I got there. I had people to talk to, and there were support groups that helped me to feel better. Doctors would visit every day, and the food was not bad and regular: three meals a day.

One of the things I started to do was barter with people for different things. I was good at this game, having played monopoly about a million times with my brother as a kid, the best negotiator always being the winner of the match. Within a short while, I had about three or four plain gold rings and some other stuff from trading tobacco and cassette tapes and such.

This hospital visit was the first time I met one of the most offensive and manipulative guys I have ever known. Adam, raised in foster care and group homes, wasn't the sharpest crayon in the box. For whatever reason, he seemed to have a large stature, though people that knew him could see he had almost no muscle and smoked a lot, so he likely had no endurance either. He was big, and he had an even bigger mouth. He would spout off that he was good enough at hockey to have made the NHL, and I bought his act of being tough one day when he nearly freaked out at me and forced me to give back some rings I had traded to him for some tobacco.

I found out later that Adam had a habit of picking fights with people, then losing badly, very badly. Then he would charge the person he had picked the fight with on an assault rap and then go to an organization called 'victim's services' and get money for being injured and traumatized. When a guy asked me why I had given his rings back when he would have told him to go stuff himself, I said that just isn't good business, when the truth was the guy freaked me out. The next day one of my doctors told me, "So Leif. We understand that you have set up a business on the ward." It just didn't seem like I should have been there. The problem was that my life outside was so empty. Getting into the hospital had lifted my spirits, and I always seemed to be looking for ways to make a buck, which I found to be fun. When I look back now, I see myself as having done more harm to others than any good to myself in that place.

At the time, I had finished just a few chapters of my first book, *Through the Withering Storm* a girl from the ward read a few chapters of it. I started to notice she liked me and we seemed to be growing closer as time went on, but then one day I asked her if she was seeing anyone and she was. The psychiatric ward being the social club that the staff tries not to let it be, I redirected my efforts to another young woman. A lot of staff have warned me about meeting members of the opposite sex while in the psychiatric ward, and it was good advice. For me, though, this was the only time that I had occasion to meet any females. I would soon learn why they warned me against it.

On one of my last days in the hospital, a psychologist gave me a test called the MMPI, or Minnesota Multi-Phasic Personality Inventory. It was a series of some 500 true or false questions, scored by computer. Just one day after I finished the test, a psychologist went through the scores for me and showed me that I appeared sane and stable and that there was no indication I was trying to fool the test or 'cheat' by answering at random. She said that this wasn't the test score of someone who needed to be in the hospital. I repeated this statement to my doctors the next day, and I was sent home. There were ways to get into support groups and counselling at the time, but I had a very serious problem. I couldn't accept being a part of groups for people who didn't function well, and I also had another problem which was that I had no means of transportation. At this point, I think it is important to note that a program was started in Edmonton a number of years later to provide low-cost bus passes to the disabled. This made a huge impact on my life and on the lives of hundreds of people.

During those last couple of days in the hospital, I became closer to the second woman I met on the ward, I even went out for a walk and brought her some flowers. It turned out that she was an independent filmmaker and had been to film school. For a while it seemed as though she was going to mentor me in the field and we made big plans. She got out of the hospital not long after I did and we ended up having a physical relationship. She was older than me. I was 25, and she was 34, and it was quite an experience to be with a woman that age.

I got her a copy of my book, and she supposedly read it then didn't contact me for a few days. Finally, I got ahold of her, and she started raving that I had stolen her manuscript, that I had taken some treasure box and some other stuff. Though I tried to sound helpful and caring, purely out of anger at the accusations, I called the police and gave them her name and address and told them she was off her medications.

I worried that she was going to try and pass my book off as her own and quite likely cause me to lose everything I had worked for and dreamed of, so right that day I set out to re-write my entire book from start to finish over the course of just a few days. This time I had some copies made and gave one of them to Debbie. From being in hospitals and living in many different places, I lost track of that book, *Through the Withering Storm*, but one day Debbie dug up her copy that I had completely forgotten about, and, thanks to her, the book has now been published. My biggest dream that I had carried with me from the time I was a very young boy and would read the titles of the classic books my mom and dad cherished, came to be.

Chapter Ten: Escape But For How Long?

Living in that small bachelor apartment had its ups and downs. It was a neat, clean, and well-kept building. Everything was new and tidy. I think I must have lived there for about two years, and near the end of that stay, one of my friends from the pool hall told me about an apartment for much cheaper. As I was on a fixed income, always trying to micro-manage each cent I had, I kept it in mind but stayed in my old place for a short while longer.

One of the things that kept haunting me was all the happy times I had in Vancouver. I had met so many interesting people while living there: actors, pilots, a nightclub owner. I did a lot of fun things like flying planes and going to parties, riding ferries and always being around such stunning scenery. I loved the idea that I was living in a real metropolitan area. In a major city, there are just so many things to do from the theaters to the beaches, and arcades and pool halls. The incredible summer weather didn't hurt either. It seemed that for the whole first ten years of me being back in Edmonton I constantly wanted to go back. It seemed each time I had the money or the desire to hitch-hike or ride the bus out there again, I would give the idea serious consideration.

One day I had gotten my disability payment, and I just decided I had enough. I got in my old Plymouth I had purchased for $75 and just took off. It was a 1,300 km journey, but I couldn't stand staying in Edmonton for even one more day. Somehow I felt I could escape my illness, go back to being young and happy and healthy, if I just made it to Vancouver. My plan was to go off my medications again and hope somehow that I would just be able to get better without them. It was a pipe dream, but it seemed so much better than just sitting there, year after year, in cold and unforgiving Edmonton. When I made it to the entrance to Jasper National Park, near the border between BC and Alberta, I felt like I was an explorer discovering a new world. The massive mountains loomed above me; and the sun was starting to come up though it was well hidden behind the high peaks. An excitement grew within me that I hadn't felt in a long time. Though I had spent most of my life in Alberta, I felt as though going down the road that would soon put me in BC was like coming home.

It was such a liberating experience for me to take off, throw some clothes and a CD player in my car and blast all my favorite music as I sang and drove. As the miles rolled away, I thought a lot about the first time I had made this trip on my own. Then, I was just 18, and I was on foot, with a few sandwiches and almost no money.

As I drove down the long highway to the Coast, I went past different places and buildings that had been significant to me since my first journey west. There was the place where a ride had let me off, leaving me to walk some 60 miles or 100 km before I got my next ride, after camping out and nearly freezing to death by the highway. There was the long high road outside of Kamloops that seemed to keep going up and up and up. There was the place where I was hitch-hiking, and a cop went past. Scared of being arrested, I hid in a ditch, because hitch-hiking was illegal. Some of the places I had been when I was coming back from Vancouver while actively suffering from my illness, I didn't see on this trip. Most likely I would never see them. I had been given bad rides and false directions so much that I could have been at the north pole for all I knew back then.

After leaving Kamloops, I picked up a hitch-hiker and we talked for quite a while as the road went past. I don't remember much about him except that when we got to Vancouver, he helped me find my way around town and when I stopped to look at my old apartment and left my car running with him in it, he didn't try to steal the thing. I dropped him off at a bus stop not long after and then went looking for a place to stay.

The first hostel I went to was the last one I had stayed in before I left Vancouver. I had left behind a ton of stuff there, including a pair of downhill skis that were a gift from my old roommate, a TV and VCR that I had bought on credit, and all the clothes and other items that I couldn't carry with me when I left. I was shuffled out the door before I could even ask about them, by some strange woman who didn't even seem to be working there. I had my doubts any of the stuff remained. Some of the people who lived there would have taken them after a few months.

I ended up going to The Jericho Beach Hostel in the west end of Vancouver. It was an old army barracks converted to dorms with a large kitchen plus a TV room and a paid cafeteria. Years ago, I had stayed there and had the time of my life playing pick-up games of soccer and baseball. On another occasion, I went to a beach party not far from there where some English girls, two guys from Ireland, and I shared poems and songs, and slept all night on the beach in sleeping bags. I was a bit worried about the ferocious Vancouver traffic, so I parked my car and took the bus everywhere. That was another thing I liked about Vancouver: there was neither any stigma nor any difficulties in riding the bus.

I don't remember too much of what I did on that trip. I think I spent a fair bit of time at the hostel, talking and playing chess and other things. I tried to get ahold of a few people I had known from living there but had no luck. I even tried to sell my car, so I could have money to stay out there. But after a few days, I realized that this was a city where you had to work hard and make good money just to make ends meet. For all its faults, Edmonton had low rents, lots of work, and I knew many people there, especially my parents who would often help me when no one else would. After three days, I hit the road for home, and since I drove in the dark and didn't know the roads, I drove at about 80 km per hour, and it took me some 18 hours to get home. I made it in my $75 car, and I didn't have to leave my parents with the job of removing and storing all my stuff from my old apartment. Also, they wouldn't have to worry themselves to death about the next time I got sick, and how they would have no way to help me.

When I got back home, I decided to be honest and tell the caretaker of my building that I was going to be late on the rent by a couple of days. The jerk came up to my apartment twenty minutes later with an eviction notice, and the rent payment wasn't even going to be late for another few days. I took my pool hall friend's advice and went and got a bachelor apartment from the place he told me was much cheaper. Now I could, at least, have a few extra bucks each month, but the apartment was tiny. It was ten feet by fifteen feet, with enough room for a desk, a table, and a bed. It wouldn't have been too bad for someone who went out a lot, but at the time I didn't go anywhere except down the street to the pool hall and sometimes the book store.

I tried to keep myself busy at this point. I went to church as much as possible. I would go to some abstinence meetings. One of my favorite things to do was to put on a radio station that had four back to back Bible study programs. I would lay down in the dark and listen to the programs for hours, night after night. I would learn later that there is a condition that people with my illness have; it is known as religious obsession, and it can cause all kinds of problems. I just didn't know any place in my life other than my church where I could associate with those who I thought were good people and wouldn't judge me. I went through a lot of times when I attended church regularly and other times when I strayed from the straight and narrow. I walked a thin line between wanting to embrace God and hiding myself away from the world.

One of the things I liked to do at that time was to walk to a local mall and go to a video store there that had movies for rent-two for a buck, and you could keep them for a week. I spent countless hours watching movies, everything from old war movies from the fifties to James Bond, the Rocky movies and on and on. If I needed money, I would find a temp agency and do a couple of hours of work, which would get me enough for a can of loose tobacco and a few groceries. The only real problem was that I had stopped seeing a psychiatrist.

This dangerous and selfish act was soon going to cause me to be sicker than I had ever been.

At the pool hall, there was this guy there who seemed friendly and I often sat with him. I would be drinking coffee, he would be drinking liquor, and he would tell me all his crime stories. After a while, he started telling me he had a connection that was getting him counterfeit five dollar bills and since he paid for everything in fives, I believed him. I asked an older friend what I should do. I wondered if the guy could bring me down with him just for sitting beside him while he passed all those fake notes, and my buddy said I should turn him in. I ended up making an anonymous call, worried out of my mind that a Hells Angels member or someone else was going to kick my door in and beat me to death for being a rat. I never heard a thing about it and time passed.

I ended up getting a three day a week janitorial job at the pool hall, and I liked it. When I was a teenager, working as a janitor in a bakery, I found that I liked the idea of working unsupervised, of cleaning things and doing a good job of it. To me, work was my life. I didn't do things for fun, I didn't believe in fun. If I rented a movie, it would be one that would teach me something useful. If I read a book, it had to contribute to my knowledge base. So I was very happy to get a job that would get me out of the house. I didn't mind mopping up a dance floor, as I walked and swung the mop, I would hum a Bruce Springsteen tune to myself and pretend I was dancing with the mop. I took a lot of satisfaction in doing the best job I could do.

Not long after that, the pizza place/bar next door had their chef come over and spy on me while I was working and was so impressed he offered me a job as a cook. I had also done this job before, and it seemed a step up from what I was doing, but a step down in pay, and I agreed to work for them. I ended up running the whole kitchen, which was easy because we only got about five or six orders on an average night. I knew a lot of the people that came and went, and we would often play cards and talk while I was working. There were a lot of interesting characters there. One was a guy, Morris, who was in his 60s and wasn't terribly sharp but very kind and helpful to his friends. One time he told me he was born in a barn and when I said I didn't believe him, he showed me his birth certificate which had a farm road address on it. Years later I was to meet his nephew, who was a prominent psychiatrist at the provincial mental hospital. I had expected to go through a grilling interview, and instead, I noticed the name and we laughed and joked about Morris, and he even confirmed that the barn story was true.

The waitress who worked there was a troubled but sweet and caring young woman named Jocelyn. The owner, Jocelyn, and I would often go for Chinese food after work. They were appalled at my fashion sense, wearing an old grey leather jacket I had bought from a thrift shop and faded old jeans. One day the owner came to me with a story that he had bought some jeans and wanted to sell them to me. They were stolen goods I found out later, but we couldn't agree on a price anyhow, so I didn't buy them.

After Jocelyn, the original waitress who worked there, there was a younger waitress who I liked spending time with named Amy. Her and I got along, but she spent a good deal of her income on pot, which I simply couldn't have in my life. I still cared about her well-being, though. One night I called her up, and she said she had a headache so I came down with some painkillers for her. Little did I know this simple act of kindness was about to put my life at risk. Inside the bar was a guy who seemed always to be spouting off, always making trouble. Rumor had it he had been kicked out of every bar in the area and was a troublesome ass.

When I got down to the bar that night, I discovered that the troublemaker had brought a knife to the bar, and had made a show of checking it with the bar staff while he was there. I picked it up to look at it; there were some interesting designs on it. It was a high-quality blade, sharpened on both sides, with what was likely a die-cast handle. I wanted to show him something with it, a little trick my brother and I used to do, and he started to freak out. I told him not to worry. I wasn't going to do anything, just a little trick and he seemed to calm down, but then he asked for the knife and wanted to throw it into the wall. I told him he couldn't do it in there, but he could do it outside if he wanted. So, I gave him the knife, and we went out to the snow-filled parking lot, and he tried to throw the weapon into a telephone pole, and the knife went some two or three feet wide of it. We went looking for it but had no luck, walking around and kicking at the snow. He left, but I kept looking.

After a few minutes, he came back and seemed to be hiding behind a fence. He said, "That was my grandfather's knife! You better find it, or I'm going to shoot you!!" I looked, and it seemed likely he did have a gun of some kind, so I ran away at an angle, hoping to make it harder for him to aim. Then he came out from behind the fence and declared that he wasn't armed. I walked in close to him and his hand, which was down at his side, came up and there was a sawed-off 20-gauge shotgun in it. I was a bit nervous, but also I was coldly calculating how close I would have to get to disarm him. I didn't get the chance.

After threatening my life, the bonehead went into the bar and threatened everyone. I'm sure his actions were a result of what I now believe was a severe mental illness, and he got beat up by the other cook. I didn't see any of this, and I was out of danger, so I decided to take off, and I called the police from a nearby restaurant. Two cops came down, and I told them the whole story, and they threatened to arrest me. Then they asked for the whole story again, and I repeated it, and I guess since I didn't make any mistakes, they began to trust a little of what I had to say. In the meantime, an undercover cop had been sent in and ended up taking the guy down. The cops took me to the west end station, and I filled out a report. While there, I met one of the Detectives that had handled the murder case involving my friend Mike. Many people wonder if it is obvious to others that they have a mental illness, they wonder especially if it is obvious to cops. These cops that took me in to make a statement were okay, but the others who threatened to arrest me had a seriously bad attitude, and I wonder if it had to do with me coming across as an impoverished and mentally ill person. Likely, they must be this way with all the different kinds of people they deal with on each call. I have had many good experiences with cops, but they always seem to treat me like garbage at first.

Not long after that incident, I quit working at that bar and went back to the whole day-labor game. I started going back to the pool hall, and my counterfeiter friend never seemed to be there, so I figured the police had caught him. Then one day he happened to come in, and I don't know if the cop gave him my name or he just figured it out, but he was aware that I had turned him in. Then he told me the police had arrested him in front of people that worked for him, and that the whole counterfeiting story was a lie. It astounded me that he wanted to threaten me and make me feel bad about something that was a total fabrication on his part. When I heard, the counterfeiting story wasn't true, I got a little more than ticked off. He had to have been a pathological liar, and I have no patience for people like that. I have often wondered if being a pathological liar is a treatable illness. I seem to have met so many. It is almost like they have formed a whole reality for themselves, (like what happens to people with psychosis), but they function, they work, they pay their bills. They just seem to have a talent for weaving webs of falsehoods wherever they go. In a way, I was lucky that this guy was a liar because no one in his group of friends thought enough of him to avenge his arrest. I got a few threats later, but didn't think much of them. I was more angry that there was a likelihood the arresting officer gave out my name to this jerk.

While I was living in my tiny basement room, a guy moved in across the hall, and we ended up being friends. He was a drywall installer and had just gotten out of prison for assault. He was another strange person, but I needed as many friends as I could get and this guy was a good friend to me. He worked a tough job and was a Christian. Although, I think that if a person is a Christian, it shouldn't be the only factor I use to decide what kind of a person they are. I have met some seriously awful ones in my life.

One of the first things we did together was go flying. There are few things I love more than flying small planes, and the building we lived in was just five minutes from Edmonton's Municipal Airport. He had been telling me that there were some swans spotted outside of St. Albert and that he wanted desperately to get a look at them, so I offered to get a plane and go and see.

The plane ride was incredible. I sat up front in the Captain's seat and did a lot of the flying, the instructor was in the co-pilot's seat and was there for any of the tricky stuff, and my friend sat in the back. By the end of the flight, my friend was so excited about the trip that he asked for forms to apply for lessons and financing for them, and I refused to let him pay for half the cost of the flight because I had so much fun back in 'the chair' again.

One time my new friend and I went out to Whyte Avenue, the 'party' district of Edmonton, and we met a couple of young women. One of them was underage, and the other was just barely legal at 18, and I ended up getting a serious crush on the one who was barely legal, who we only knew as Silver. She had the potential of being somebody. She had won academic awards in high school, had scholarships, and was an accomplished women's basketball player. She had just gone down the wrong path, and I felt somehow that I could rescue her. She was a drug user, mostly pot and ecstasy. The feelings I had for her were so strong; I was nearly willing to risk everything and use drugs with her, hoping that doing so could make us closer. Luckily, I didn't. We had some fun times; going for car trips and hanging out at coffee shops. I even played the odd game of basketball with her. Then she went away for a while and left some stuff at my place, and when she came back to get it, she was with some guy who she said was just a friend but must have also had feelings for her. I told her that if she ever needed it, she could stay with me and I will never forget how she said: "I would definitely live with you." I felt as though I had finally climbed the peak, that at last my life wouldn't be so lonely, but sadly, I was never to see her again. With what I was about to go through, maybe that was for the best.

Chapter Eleven: Regulation Jail Cell

It was kind of harsh living for as long as I did in that ten foot by fifteen-foot apartment. For a good part of that time, I would make frequent trips to the mall and eat a bunch of donuts I got from the grocery store then buy whatever fattening foods were on sale and pretty much ignore all the fresh produce. I started gaining a lot of weight, but I didn't notice because I had no scale and didn't go to the pool as much back then as I do now. I had stopped caring much about my looks until a friend suggested to me that I try abstinence groups for people who had food as their addiction. I asked him how he knew I needed such a place and he replied with honesty that he could tell just by looking at me. All the while I had developed one addiction or another I wished that there was an ongoing support program for people with schizoaffective disorder. I think the reason there isn't any groups like that could be the stigma, and it could be that until recently people with illnesses like mine mostly weren't expected to recover.

I ended up going to the overeating groups, and I got a lot out of them. Like other meetings I went to, though, I didn't see the point of working through the program laid out for self-improvement. I just thought that the object was to quit the behavior, while it was more about building up morals and honesty so you wouldn't even think of engaging in your self-destructive behavior. I went to three or four meetings and then stopped and spent the next six months starving myself. It worked: I lost a lot of weight, but I had missed the point of the program entirely. That could be why that for some time, until the last 10 years, I seemed to move from one addictive behavior to another.

The other problem that surfaced right around that time was that I was finding I never had enough energy, that I was sleeping too much, eating too much and not being able to get anything done. The worst part of it was that often I would make plans with my dad or friends and they would come to get me. In the time from me talking to them on the phone to the time they got there, I would fall asleep and was so tired (often from staying up all night) that I wouldn't get up even when they banged on my window or honked their horn. I decided that the problem was with my medication, and I thought things would be okay if I just lowered one of them by 50%. I would still be taking everything, just a little less of one.

Many times, while I lived in my ten foot by fifteen foot cell, I would end up so far into a depression from loneliness that I would end up calling the Alberta Hospital Crisis Team or the local suicide helpline. I would talk with them for a while, feel better, then hang up and it wouldn't be too long until I was feeling horrible again. I needed to have some hope that I could grow past my illness, some way of structuring my life to get me the medications and support I needed for recovery. After my friend, the drywall installer, had moved out of the building, I was mostly just interacting with people in chat rooms on the computer. I would talk with some of them on the phone, but I never met any of them in person. Back when the Internet was just starting, I read an advice column that suggested if you are socially insecure you should go on the Internet. It is funny now to understand that a lot of people who write these articles and columns have no actual training in the field of psychology or psychotherapy; they simply have a knack for writing articles. Most magazines require you to give advice for the article to fit the magazine. As I look back now, suggesting I do something so isolating like letting the computer take over my social life would be the worst thing I could do.

As time passed from the time I cut back my medication, I started to grow a little worse mentally each day. It was an imperceptible but very real progression. Because of the fact that it was now over seven years since I had first ruined my credit rating when I had traveled to the US at age 19, I started applying for credit cards and getting them. I started with a department store card, put small purchases on it and paid them back, then tried for lines of credit and major credit cards, and I got them. At the time, I wasn't working, but I had been offered a job writing comedy skits for a small television network in Ontario, which never materialized. I just knew what to put on the applications and ended up getting myself in deep financial trouble sooner than I expected.

This church had a lot of strange ideas. Some of the more traditional people in it didn't go to movies, and the church forbade dancing, along with alcohol, tobacco, and even jewelry (though firearms and hunting were just fine.) I was glad to be rid of all but a few close friends from there, and, after meeting some very cool young women, I started attending a Catholic Bible study and was so impressed by the way they looked at worship I made a decision to become a Catholic. It wasn't something that happened overnight. I had supposed that I would eventually go back to the Pentecostal Church once I was over being upset with this dork and hopefully, he wouldn't be there. I thought I would just be able to go back to having a few friends and a rewarding spiritual life. Before that happened, though, I wanted to keep my faith nurtured, and so as these two young women offered, I attended a Catholic Bible study with them.

One of the two women was single and had been in Air Cadets. I had a bit of romantic interest in her, but I am the kind of person to take things pretty slow. I had only ever had one girlfriend, and I made sure we were close before I revealed my feelings to her which I felt was a better way to do things. I don't have much knowledge of forming relationships, but I have had a few female friends in my life who were kind of cool, and friendship is something I don't like to jeopardize. The funny thing is that quite often I will admit that I am bipolar before admitting that I am interested in a potential girlfriend. At that time, my mental health was stable, though declining. I even had a car and a cell phone. It is so hard to describe to people what it means to be bipolar but to be in remission. The ravages of the illness don't just affect you when you are ill. They can make life pretty bleak in other ways. Luckily, I was reasonably free of those feelings, for which I thank my anti-depressants, but I was still under the curse of living alone.

Living alone is something that no person with a mental illness should do. There are times when I like my solitude, but when it is forced on you 24 hours a day, and you have a hard time making friends, it can be a hardship. Add in a roller coaster of emotions, even a medication-treated roller coaster, and the fact that my apartment was 10 feet by 15 feet-the mix can be lethal. Twice in the same year, a few years before that, I had to be hospitalized in an attempt to get me living more like an average person: sleeping during the night and getting my medications at the proper times.

The Catholic Bible study was a lot of fun. The people there were around my age and did things for work that were interesting. The young woman I wanted to get to know better was named Carol. She did seem to kind of like me, and as we had a similar background from being in Cadets, she had suggested I might like going and instructing a summer camp course called 'boot camp' that was being run by the Knights of Columbus. Then one day at the study, they showed a video of a man who was an incredible intellectual, talking about how he became a Catholic and all at once I saw some kind of beauty and perfection in the Catholic Church. I was deeply moved and started to learn more and more about the Catholic Faith, a good deal of it from the website of this same person from the video.

When fall came, I got a friend to sponsor me to take the class to become a Catholic, and he was incredibly helpful in many ways. The thing that eases my conscience about not completing the course was that my friend's dad had bipolar, and when I started getting sick he understood what was happening. I did some strange things aside from slimming down from just about obese to dangerously skinny. One of the strange things I did was I went to the Catholic Church near my apartment and somehow felt a holiness, a glow of who God was. I walked around the building, praying what is called the stations of the cross, then I sat down and closed my eyes, and I saw a rough image of what looked like a black and grey eclipse. The sun seemed to come out in Israel, where Christ was born. This vision appeared to be a divine revelation that Christ was going to be born again and come back to complete the prophecy of the New Testament. I was so convinced that this was true that I told my Priest about it and he didn't know how to respond.

One Sunday after I went to Mass, I crossed the street to buy some matches, and when I was told they didn't have any, some guy in the store lashed out in anger at me. Being in a poor mental state, I argued back. He told me to get out of the kiosk, and I did, and he and another guy followed me out, and I gave them both the finger. I wish that incident was the worst that had happened to me, but a few days later I went to my parent's house to pay them back some money, and while walking to their place from the nearby bank machine, I crossed the street and a car had to stop for me. Then I went on walking across, and after going a few yards, I heard someone yelling at me. It was the driver of the car, and he was hopping mad. He came running after me, knocked me down and punched me in the face a bunch of times. Ever since I was tiny, I have never been bothered by a few punches. I got a lot of them at home and school, from my brother or a bully or whatever. It just amazed me that this guy wanted to harm me just because he had to step on his brake for a second.

When I went to my parent's house after that, it left my mom in a terrible state to see me all bruised and battered. My dad also must have been worried sick. The blows had swollen my whole face, and I had two black eyes. I was starting to realize that something was wrong, I just had no idea what to do about it. I had little control especially since some of my old delusions were coming back. One of the worst things about the kind of delusions I had was that they were a false reality that seemed so much better than what I was living. I believed a lot of weird things, and soon my behavior was just as strange. These delusions usually started with thoughts that forced their way into my mind. In the delusions, there was an evil woman trying to torture me for whatever reason, or some VIP who was running a multi-billion-dollar corporation that included the assets of most of the world that was waiting for me to regain my fortune. It was enough to give a person an ulcer, having no money in reality, but being bombarded with thoughts of great riches just around the corner.

I don't know why I didn't have a full realization then that I was delusional. When I am on medications and understand that my delusional thoughts are false creations of a mind that has a chemical imbalance, I can recognize that I go through a pattern. First, I would go off my medications. Second, I would get angry that higher forces and powers are playing with my head. Third, I would inescapably end up in a psychiatric ward or a mental hospital.

No matter how much I hated it when I was sick and ended up in a psychiatric ward or a mental hospital, the psychiatric ward or hospital would get me better. It wasn't a pleasant place to be. Inside the ward I was confined to there were many people who were very seriously ill and it was not only difficult to interact with them, it was difficult to deal with my own symptoms, which at times didn't seem like delusions, they seemed very real to me. Part of my mind was on overload with all of the false thoughts and disturbing thoughts. Part of me knew that I desperately needed treatment.

On this occasion, I went to see my medical doctor, and when I went into the examining room he got a phone call, left, and was gone for a while. I went out and opened the only closed door, and there he was, talking to members of the crisis team who were from the hospital. They had been following me around for a while, trying to possibly wait for a time to intervene to have me admitted to the hospital. I ended up chatting with them, and a friendly pair of ambulance drivers took me to the hospital. The paramedics were even good enough to join me in a cigarette before leaving for 'the bin.'

The next few days went well. My doctor seemed to think that I hadn't been taking any of my medications and started me on a new circuit of drugs which didn't seem as beneficial to me as the last ones were. I liked the idea of just taking one pill and left it at that. This visit I was there for less time than I had ever spent in the hospital, and my doctor seemed like a nice guy. I got along well with the other staff, and patients on the ward that time. One of them had invented his own board game, we played it, and it was fun. There was another guy who I hung around with a lot who liked card tricks and was always getting the staff to pick up more cards for him and more sesame seed snacks. I have always had a strong suspicion that he was making some form of alcohol out of them but never confirmed it.

After a week, I got a pass to go home for a couple of days, and I went and got my car and drove it back to the hospital and parked it in a farmer's field. It was difficult to operate a car well when you are on a new medication, but I got through okay. I was released after another few days there, and I thought all was fine. It was nearing the beginning of summer, and I felt good. Little did I know I could never have been more wrong about what was about to happen to me.

Chapter Twelve: Mind Numb and Delusional

Newly released from the hospital after just a short stay, I made the decision to take things into my own hands because I didn't like the side effects of the new pill I had been put on. I did one of the worst things a person could do who is on medications: I went back to my old pharmacy and got my old meds and went back to taking them with my doctor having no knowledge of the switch.

After that point, it seemed that everything happened in a frenzy. Now and then, friends would drop by, or neighbors would come by with food or for a visit and they were appalled at my condition. I was way underweight, and horribly delusional. None of them knew what to do for me. I had one friend that lived way on the south side of Edmonton, and I can remember going for a drive with him and not making any sense. I kept on babbling about being a University student (I was taking a University correspondence course) and how I could communicate across great barriers and accomplish things that would change the world. Everything I did like that later became such a shame and an embarrassment to me; the incidents burned their way into my memory. It didn't help that this particular friend was a joker and told me in detail how he and his wife had a good laugh while they played and re-played some of my confusing phone messages. What had happened was I would call people up and talk like some slow-witted person for no real reason. I sent confusing messages to people over the Internet and even phoned up my former Cadet Sergeant, which I wish I hadn't done.

Then there was another guy I had known since high school. I had called his wife a couple of times because I knew she wasn't working but staying home taking care of their baby, and he must have thought I was hitting on her or something. He was one of the people I knew who blamed all my problems on a harsh upbringing, particularly the fact that my Dad didn't treat me too well. I had a chemical imbalance in my nervous system. My treatment as a child had nothing to do with my illness. After finally talking to this former friend directly, he hung up on me and blocked my number.

I would still lay in the dark in the evenings and listen to either music or Bible study radio programs. Somehow, my mind manufactured the idea that one of my engineer friends, and a young woman I had delusional thoughts about, could change the channels on the radio by satellite to show me they were supporting my efforts. In my head, I was linked to Jesus and God and all the wealthy people and leaders in the world. I believed that they had a special microchip in my head and a listening device in my dental filling. Strangely, I had lengthy and sensible explanations for these ideas, and they were possible according to modern technology, though incredibly improbable considering my situation. The problem was that they were inventions of my mind. I was also convinced there was someone outside my window watching me: it was a pair of workers from the provincial mental hospital who were waiting for their chance to convince me or force me to go back to the hospital.

The final straw came when I walked out of my apartment one day, and the front door was broken, and wouldn't open. I went into a panic. I thought that someone had planted a bomb in the building and sealed the exits to kill everyone. I ran around the building trying to alert everyone, then went out the back door. I went to the caretaker's suite and buzzed "dot dot dot dash dash dash dot dot dot," the sequence for 'save our souls' or SOS in Morse code. The caretaker stuck her head out the window and wasn't too happy. I told her about the so-called 'emergency,' and she went back inside. Then some guy in an older car pulled up, and I thought he was going to get blown to pieces if he stopped his car, so when he opened his door I kicked it shut. I kicked it a few times, and he got mad as a hatter. Then everybody started coming: cops, crisis workers, ambulances. I ended up waiting in the caretaker's office as they came. I sat there for a while and talked to the nurses from the mental health crisis team and the whole while this cop stood in the next room staring at me and saying nothing. It angered me, so I went to walk up to him and shake his hand, hoping to break the tension barrier. He looked at me with disgust and said that he didn't shake hands. Of all the things that happened that day, he was the only one who showed blatant disrespect.

Soon, after bumming a cigarette, and being strapped into an ambulance chair, I was taken back to the hospital. At the time, the Prince of Wales (Prince Charles) was in Canada, and I had an interesting talk with one of the ambulance drivers who had stood guard for him as part of his duties as a member of the Reserves. We talked about some interesting things we had in common and he expected I would be admitted quietly to the hospital and all would go well. It didn't work that way.

The paramedic I had conversed with brought me to the admissions desk and talked about how I was a good guy and had behaved myself. Then I found out that Dr. Murphy, oversaw admitting and something clicked. He had been my doctor when I was in the hospital during the previous stay, and I didn't like him too much. I made some racist remarks about him being a drunk and started to back out of the admitting office. My paramedic friend tried to talk me into going back, but then for some reason, I just bolted running as fast as possible away from everyone. I thought, for some reason, that if I made it to the chapel, I could claim sanctuary. I was severely beaten and manhandled by the staff when they caught up with me. They also strapped me to a gurney, with the additional insult of being pumped full of whatever medications they gave me.

The delusions in my head were horrible at that point, and it seemed that my doctor had no interest in doing anything about them. A few days after I got there he came to my room to see me, and right in front of me gave the head nurse permission to lock me into the isolation room for the slightest thing.

I don't know if I can really blame the people in the hospital for the way I was treated, I was very sick. One of my delusions was that I was going to be the next King of England. It sounds preposterous, but when it is broken down, it almost makes sense (provided it isn't the words of a mentally ill person). Not long before this incident, my Dad had a visit from his brother who lived in Denmark. My Uncle had spent 40 years in the Danish Navy and was knighted for his outstanding service. On a recent visit, he had brought some things from Denmark for us, and one of them was an ancient-looking book with hand-carved wooden covers. I didn't understand Danish, but my Dad said it traced our blood lines all the way back to the 12th century. If you can go that far back, one can use their bloodlines to prove relations to anyone. Now, remembering that I was delusional about some wealthy young woman trying to make me into something, it wasn't a far stretch for me to be deluded that I had a lot of money and power. Though fictional, I had reason to believe there was some money somewhere in my family. In the grand scope of my misfiring mind, I was heir to untold sums of money and power. Some proof seemed to exist that I could be declared royalty in one way or another. Take this delusion of power and fame, and you have a short "hop-skip and jump" to me being named King. It's preposterous, really, but that was how messed up my thoughts were.

As Dr. Murphy requested, I was put into the isolation room many times. One time I was put there because a staff member decided he wasn't going to hand me a tray for supper. He then put me in a painful arm lock and had me forcibly confined to the room. They didn't need a reason. They didn't even need two people or even one doctor to decide I should be isolated. They simply threw me in and locked the door. Sometimes, I would be in the isolation room for days. I would just go completely nuts. I would kick the door and scream. I had been given a bottle to urinate in, and I would fill it up and then find a way to splash it under the door so the staff members would unknowingly step in it. That must have ticked them off because after a month or so of me being there they had put a special rubber stopper under the door so that no one could do that.

My illness also made me think people in the ward were people I knew that had changed their appearance by makeup or surgery and were running this place so they could torture me. There was one psychology student who was kind to me even though I kept thinking she was someone else.

It seemed there was a revolving door of staff and patients there, for all but me. I was there for a long time. The main reason for this was that often I would go to the desk to ask about something with regards to medications or the like, and the staff would say to me, "You have to talk to your doctor." At one point my doctor didn't see me for more than a month, so I told the staff, "The Doctor never sees me, he is incompetent." And they kept telling me to tell him that to his face. So one day I did.

"'Doctor Murphy," I said, "Your nursing staff is cruel and hateful. I want another doctor and a different nurse. The nurse is incompetent and so are you!"

"Get out!" was all he said, and aside from bumping into him in the parking lot, he never spoke to me for the next five months I was a patient on that ward.

I don't know what he did to my medications, but whatever it was they weren't working. I remember I would wake up, roll a cigarette, go into the TV room and watch the news, and I kept on hearing and seeing the guy on the TV talk about me. He would say things like, "Brought to you by Leif Gregersen." Or, "Leif

Gregersen is to be told he has a billion dollars." I would quickly finish my smoke, then head back to my room and roll another one. When I got up to three or four, the TV would stop talking to me, and I would feel much closer to some form of sanity.

So many things happened in the time I was there. One day a woman came in who looked kind of old though she was only 41. I was just about 30 at the time, and for whatever reason, I thought she was the young woman who had taken control of my brain through a microchip or a relative of that same young woman. She had quite an abrasive attitude, but I just kept doing nice things for her and eventually she warmed up to me. We would talk a lot, write long letters to each other and became good friends, but, for some reason, the staff had decided that we shouldn't associate. They kept telling her to stay away from me, but up until the time the doctors took her to another ward, she was a great encouragement to me to get through all the garbage life was throwing at me.

Another person who was essential to me getting through that incredible ordeal of pain and mental 'storms' was my dad. He had gone as far as contacting the newspapers to get someone to come down and bring to light the way I was being treated. My father's actions were no delusion either: there were periods when my dad would come to visit, and he would hear me screaming in the isolation room, or other times when I would have black eyes and other marks on my body. Once a patient had tried to sever my jugular vein and in doing so left these horrible scratch marks down my neck. It was getting ridiculous. And all the while the staff were looking for ways to get me into legal trouble. Their first gambit was to try and turn me in for fraud because I had credit cards. Then some guy decided to pick a fight with me, and the staff did everything they could to try and get the guy to charge me with assault.

All this was reprehensible, but perhaps the worst of it was that I wasn't allowed to use the phone at all. I could pace the halls, go nuts in the side room, or smoke myself to death, but I wasn't allowed any contact with the outside world. It scares me now just to think of it. That place couldn't have been a worse torture chamber for a person who is ill and vulnerable.

Chapter Thirteen: Finding a Way Through

There was a lot of bad and some good that happened when I was in the lock-up ward. There was one small guy who was a loyal friend and he was always playing pranks on the staff. One of the things he liked to do was hide under the hollow, wooden coffee tables they had in the ward. The staff counted the patients every half hour, so they would come up one short and go into a panic until my friend came out from under a coffee table laughing himself sick.

For a good part of my stay in that awful place, I was also friends with a guy named John Lifton. I can remember telling him that I had gone to church with the son of a political candidate, and that I didn't like him, and I would do anything to see him fail. He told me his dad was one of the Directors of the political party this guy was running with. Meeting this guy in my church was the worst experience I had ever had there. After I had met him, I swore I would never go there again. I like to think it was indirectly the hand of God that did it, but just a few short months after I left the church, there was some infestation, perhaps termites, that caused the whole place to be condemned and torn down right to the basement.

Before I knew who he was, I had noticed that the unnamed son of the political leader from the church was always getting praise and preference in everything he did. It was troubling, but I put my ego aside and decided I would talk to him and give him a chance. I went up to him and asked what he did, and he said he was a stock broker. I had recently made some investments and was thinking of taking the securities course. I thought this might be an excellent opportunity to get this guy on my side, so I asked him a question or two about what he liked in the markets lately, and he looked down his nose at me and said, "I don't even think about work on the weekend." The way he said it seemed as though he was trying to show how he was a Christian and didn't work on Sundays and I was some infidel daring to even speak to him. I tried to talk with him further, but, after insulting me once more, he invited me to a party at his house for some strange reason. I went, but when I got there, he took up half an hour praying in front of everyone that he receive protection from a guy who had come into the church not knowing anything about faith and asked him for help. I couldn't imagine anyone doing anything more despicable or hypocritical. Not to mention that he was trying to make himself out to be something he wasn't.

It is disturbing how quickly my mind degenerated into the state it was in while I was in the Provincial Mental Hospital. During my extended Hospital stay, John Lifton became something of a good friend. I learned that previously he had been in the forensic part of the hospital for 30 days or so and that he was in no shape to face the world when they let him out, so they locked him up in another part of the hospital. I didn't resent this so much with John, but the non-forensic part of the hospital got a lot of the overflow of patients from forensics. Add that to the figure a doctor once gave me that 80% of the people in forensics are convicted murderers, and you get something of an interesting mix of individuals.

Some of the people there were scary to be around. One of them was a guy who drove a truck for a living, and anytime you sat near him to chat for a little while he would start saying things like he was a filmmaker and his plans to 'blow the lid off' the conspiracy were what got him in there. I once looked at the paper he carried with him for notes and it was all scrambled with phone numbers and names and stuff, none of it in any order, just haphazardly scrawled in wherever he found space to do so. How he managed to buy his truck and run it as a business, I will never know. What I did know is that he gave away to people what must have been at least $500 and possibly $1,000 of cigarettes, and sometimes when he talked to you, he would go off on tangents and then get outraged and start yelling if you didn't agree with him. It was sad because he could have been somebody if he was either properly treated or if he properly used his medications or if he perhaps never had a mental illness.

One of the more heart-wrenching things about ending up in the hospital is that it seemed that there was no way I could get any better, even enough so I could go a year without being thrown back in there. I had been on another ward twice in the same year a short time previous to being put in the lock-down ward. One of the visits was actually kind of a nice one. I had a doctor that would see me every day and I had a friend who I hung out with a lot. His name was Nick, and he was a pathological liar who was so skilled in his imaginations that very rarely did anyone catch him in a lie, and when they did he would go right back to lying again. He had told me he was in cadets and that he was a pilot and all kinds of things like that. He even read parts of my first book. He also said he had slept with a young woman I used to work and go to school with-anything that would make him look like more than he was. One of the amazing things about his lies was that he somehow seemed to believe them, and he had an incredible capacity to make other people believe the garbage he would dish out.

Nick and I did a lot of things that summer when I was in the hospital. We borrowed bikes from the recreation centre and rode them around the back highways when we had permission to leave our ward. We played a lot of badminton. Nick led me to believe that he was from a wealthy family and that he would have a high-paying job for me plus the use of a truck when I was out of the hospital. Then when I left the hospital, I lost all contact with him. His phone number no longer worked, and I didn't have his address. I even tried calling his dad who, understandably, wouldn't give out any information. Still, that was actually an enjoyable stay in the hospital, much different from the five months I spent in the locked ward a few years later.

As far as my time in the locked ward goes, I made friends with a few people. However, a couple of the staff seemed to dislike me a great deal. One of the most annoying things the treatment team used to do was to come to everyone's room and shine a flashlight in your face every few minutes while you were trying to sleep. It made it nearly impossible to sleep, and when you are a heavy smoker, and they close the smoking room all night, not sleeping gets to be a severe discomfort. One or two times I bitched at this one guy on staff who was overweight. Just to piss him off even more, I would sometimes call him the "stay-puff marshmallow man." My delusions had me convinced he was a member of a motorcycle gang and did violent, awful things to people in the hospital.

As mentioned, they put me in the isolation room often, which used to upset me so much I could swear I was getting ulcers. I know that I did end up with severe acid reflux so bad I was in great pain. It doesn't seem like that serious a condition, but in fact, acid reflux killed my mother at the age of 63. Her breathing passage simply became unable to function and she passed away. Being put in isolation (often just because they felt like doing so), I did anything I could to get back at them; from karate-kicking the door to my personal favorite, taking the bare mattress they left in the room and propping it up against the wall and hiding behind it. Whoever was watching me then had to come in and confiscate the mattress, and they would leave me with nothing but a thing called a 'strong sheet' and the cold tile floor. One time I asked to use the toilet that was attached to the room, which was locked, and the guy I called 'stay-puff' decided this would be a good time to get back at me for whatever I had done to him. We fought, and I grabbed his 'life call' button, which was an alarm button all the staff carried around their necks, and pressed it just to see what would happen. Lo and behold, a siren went off, and about 20 staff members came sprinting into my little isolation room. It was a good thing, too, because 'Stay-Puff' was so angry with me he balanced himself on the backs of my knees; I tried to tell him I had injured my knees and he was causing me further serious injury, but still I had to wrestle with him to stop him from doing it.

There was another incident during that stay with a different staff member, the one who used to get John his library materials. I was not in the greatest of moods, and this particular psychiatric aide was gently playing guitar in the main lobby of the ward. I got mad at him because his playing was going through my head like a nail and I demanded he stop playing. He told me if I didn't stop pointing my finger at him he would break it off. I ceased pointing the finger, but I didn't stop bitching, and he said, "That's it, Leif! If I ever see you outside of this place I'm going to beat the shit out of you." He was such a scumbag. Once, I got him back with a vengeance, though. I was walking up and down the hall one day for exercise, and when I was in the women's part of the ward, I caught him staring in the room of a female patient who was most likely undressing, and scared the crap out of him by yelling at him. That felt good.

One of the people I regret being angry with was the ward social worker. It was for a legitimate reason that I was upset, but I did some mean things to her. When I got to the ward, I had no change of clothes. I had no books or computer, not even a simple change of socks. I did have money in the bank, and several credit cards but the staff took all that away from me and the ability to go home just to get a change of clothes. One day I was asked to go see the ever-absent psychiatrist, and I went to his office and sat down, and he said, "Do you know what this is?" He pointed at a paper on his desk.

"No, what is it?" I replied.

"This is a certificate of incompetency." I wanted to say that if it were for him, I would sign it gladly, but it was actually, to my surprise, for me. This document stated that I was no longer competent to handle money and that a public trustee would now handle my affairs. They had decided this because I wasn't working and had credit card debt. The part they didn't mention was that all the cards were in good standing and that the only reason I didn't have a job was because I was in the hospital. I was out of my mind, but that also had to do with my never present psychiatrist. This declaration was pure spite.

The way the Social Worker came in was that I kept trying to get her to get me some money from one of my cards or the bank or whatever, so I could get someone to buy me cigarettes. I hounded her, too. Then, later on during my stay in the ward, while I was still on poor terms with her, my sister and her moved all my possessions to a storage shed. No small job if you know what a hoarder I used to be and how little space I had for a couple of tons of books and other things. I ran into her shopping for groceries and apologized to her. She was kind enough to say that she never held things like that against people. She must have had the biggest heart in that whole complex.

I stayed friends while I was in there with a high school friend who worked at a fast food restaurant with me way back when we were 15. At one point he and his fiancée mailed me a 'care' package that had a can of tobacco and some chocolate bars and such in it. Aside from my daily visits from my dad, that was all the outside contact I had. One time I was allowed to use the phone and I called up a lawyer I had dealt with in the past and told him I wanted to sue the History Channel for using my name in their broadcasts. I didn't speak to him, but I left the message on his answering machine and then never talked to him again despite repeated attempts. One time I even got his secretary and she got really mad because I told her that I didn't care if he was in a meeting, I needed to talk to him. She ended up yelling at me, and the lawyer never returned my call.

One of the terrible things I remember about that place was that one time I was sleeping and then woke up needing to use the bathroom, and as I walked out to the hallway for some reason, my unsound mind saw a pattern, something dark and evil in the linoleum on the floor. It had to do with Hitler and WW II which I had studied extensively for a long time in younger days. It seemed to grow and evolve and spread out over Europe and the world. It was like I saw pure evil, and the feeling went right down to the pit of my stomach. I felt like all was lost in the world, like I had failed in everything. The horrible truth was that I was a hated, lonely, sick, screwed up and broke person. I almost wish I could go back to that time and change things, but now I have recovered from that horrible state. I still need a doctor's supervision and heavy medications for my affliction, but now I can see in some way that perhaps it was something I had to go through for something greater-that it would fundamentally change who I was to become. Some divine purpose, perhaps, and it has nothing to do with me being rich or powerful. I think it has to do more with just my voice, my words, my ordeal.

Chapter Fourteen: Release, On Conditions

On the ward was an incredible doctor who had immigrated from the former Soviet Union. He was kind and knew his stuff and didn't mind spending a session discussing Russian Literature or modern psychiatric methods on the other side of the globe. He had been a soldier in the Russian Army and, despite his kind demeanor and gentle voice, he was a bit scary to deal with when I was hallucinating and delusional. I went to see him one time when Dr. Murphy was away, and he saved my life. He had me transferred out of the lock-up ward and into an open one. Dr. Murphy tried to block him from doing so, but the Russian doctor's word stood. I was free of the pit at last.

On the new ward, upstairs from the lock-up, there were a few people my age, the nurses were much kinder, and there wasn't even an isolation room. There was a doctor better than any I had experienced, named Dr. Li. He was Japanese I believe, and as far as I was concerned, he was a rejuvenating breath of fresh air compared to Dr. Murphy and his flying circus of psychiatric treatment. Dr. Li would spend an entire half hour with each person under his care that needed it, each and every day. I remember going into his office one time, feeling very depressed and he told me:

"Leif, you're a nice person and people like you. Things are going to get better. You have a long life ahead of you." He always seemed to have these little encouragements for me, small chains of words that brought me back to the idea that I could still accomplish something with my life, I could still see Europe again and do the things I wanted to do.

For a while, I was given a job in an occupational therapy shop on hospital grounds that dismantled electrical meters for recycling, and it paid $1.50 an hour. It seemed like nothing, but it helped pass the time and helped me focus on something other than the fact that I had just spent five months of my life in the inner ring of hell. One day a bolt or a metal chip flew into my eye, and I got it out and went back to the ward for a scheduled appointment with Dr. Li, and he got out his stethoscope and examined me right there. The first warning flag a person has to watch out for in a Psychiatrist is one who doesn't remember the time they spent in medical school, or worse yet, one who refuses to remember because they feel it is beneath them. The doctor I had for many years, Dr. Bishop, who wrote the foreword for my first book, *Through The Withering Storm* was incredible. He would counsel me all the time with regards to medical advice and treatment, and I think being able to do that adds a lot to the respect a patient has towards a psychiatrist's opinion of what needs to happen for their mental health.

When I was 19, and in that same hospital, I had just done serious damage to my knees and could barely walk. My doctor told me that he didn't deal with those sorts of problems. I fought to see a doctor, an MD, and I don't remember if they had one. When I was there for my six-month visit, they did have an MD for that sort of stuff. At 19, after complaining for weeks of the pain and my inability to walk, I was told an appointment was made for me to see an orthopedic surgeon. They gave me a date which was a couple of months in the future. I waited and waited, and when my appointment was near, a nurse told me, "Oh, I didn't think you still wanted that. I canceled the appointment." Meanwhile, I suffered, thinking I could never get any treatment or help for my injury.

I often wonder if that appointment could have saved me years of pain and inactivity because some nurse felt she was a better judge of my pain than I was. If I had been dealing with Dr. Li or Dr. Bishop, I would have gotten far better care. It is scary to think of how quickly some doctors can skate past the gates of competency-especially in the mental health system.

After being transferred to Dr. Li's care, my new doctor told me that I should be able to leave the hospital in a month. The only sad part of that was that I had no idea that I was going to enter a much different world than the one I had left six months before. It was September 2001 when I went to that ward. 9/11 was about to change everything I ever knew. Not a total change, but everything was going to be just a little different, and some things were going to change drastically.

I was watching TV on September 11th, 2001 when the planes hit the two towers and the Pentagon. Having been a bit of a military-obsessed person, I remember a few specific things crossing my mind. I knew it was a suicide bomber, someone who had taken control of the planes. The fact that they were good enough at flying to hit those towers dead-on meant they were likely pilots. I remember feeling worse for the

3,000 people that died in those attacks than I felt about the possibility of a war coming. I didn't try and do any forecasting from what I remember, as a lot of my life near that point in time had been spent worrying about myself and the 10 foot by 10 foot cell I was in and how I was going to get out of it.

What I do remember, aside from the candlelight vigil the people at the hospital set up on the front steps of the building I was in, was that I didn't think this event would lead to global war or nuclear war. All my life I had been terrified of the idea of nuclear war perhaps because it left no chance of survival for anyone-not even an iota. The 'nuclear winter' and hydrogen bombs, and the resulting degeneration of society back to the stone age (if that many people survived) scared the life out of me. I think my fear was so acute because it is one thing for a person to die, but for everyone to die would be devastating: my parents, my sister, and brother, my uncles, and aunts across the Atlantic in Denmark. I could never have imagined anything worse, but this act on 9/11, to me seemed to be something that would trigger retaliations, but not a global war. If a war came of it, it wouldn't be one I could go to anyhow, not with my age, not with my mental illness records.

I didn't know too much about the events surrounding 9/11. I didn't know that the government had closed the border. I had little idea of the impact of the shutting down of all air traffic and the fact that the USA was likely on DEFCON 2 at the time. I do remember listening to the morning show on the radio, and they ran the show late to give any breaking news, and some bonehead called in and told them they should get off the air and play some music.

When the day ended, I was still a resident of a mental hospital and all I could think about was doing what I could to get out of there. Luckily, a couple of weeks before I was put in this new ward I had been put on some medications that started to work for me. What bothers me the most is that it was the same medication that I was taking before I was put in there, but I was willing to eat dried shit if it would get me out of that hospital. It did start to work, and I don't know how or why but as I got better and better, people would just look at me and somehow they could tell I wasn't sick anymore. It was near that time that Dr. Li had discussed discharging me from the hospital. I wanted to get out of there at any cost, and somehow I did.

The social worker 'found' me a room for rent in the basement of a lady that I suspect was a little more than a friend of his. It wasn't even a room: it was just some space in her basement that she had partially walled off with an office partition. Living there, though I had some more freedom, was one of the worst experiences I have ever had. The first thing I wanted to do was go to my storage closet and get my computer and a TV, so I would have something to occupy my time. She did drive me there but my new roommate and my new landlady both refused to help me with anything, and I ended up destroying a brand new $300 computer monitor. The worst part about that place though, was the food. We were paying $600 a month (and at the time my income was $800), and that was supposed to include food. I can't believe how stupid or cruel (or both) this woman was.

She would bring down a plate or two of boiled potato slices, no meat but a little thin gravy and call that supper. Then she would say we could put it in the microwave for two seconds if we wanted. It was criminal.

One day her sister came over and decided to do some laundry and later the landlady came down and started screaming about one of us running the washer with hot water. She screamed in my face, "Who did this? Who did this?" I said, "Your sister."

She replied, "Oh, my sister!" and didn't even apologize. In fact, she looked at me like I was the one who had done it and was lying.

Another time she came downstairs and screamed in my face that she couldn't rent out more rooms because I smell and she said, "You're a pig! You're a dirty pig!" when in fact I took a shower every single day. My shoes might have been a bit smelly, but no one deserves an insult/assault like that. I called the police on her.

The cop came and talked to her first, then came down and I calmly explained what she did, and the cop said, "Well, you're not telling the whole story. I'll say this, though. If I have to come here again tonight, I'm taking you to Alberta Hospital."

It was amazing. Not only was this woman making a fortune renting a 'room' but she could go mad on a power trip and never have to face any consequences because she was 'helping people' or even 'helping sick people.' I stayed with my parents for a few days. Then a different social worker at the mental health clinic found me the place I ended up living at for fifteen years. Because of having a stable environment, proper medication, support, and encouragement, I have not had to go back to the hospital or any psychiatric ward since (aside from the time I worked on one as a Security Guard).

Moving into where I would live long-term had a lot of advantages over any place I had been before. It was a multi-house group home with staff on duty, but if you are put in one of the outside houses as I had been, you live in a comfortable house and get along as best you can. You still get meals at the main house where the staff stays for the most part. The meals were of a decent quality, and there is a sense you live in sort of a 'community' where everyone is either trained to deal with people with mental illnesses or has one themselves. In this situation, a person feels a lot more at home and can go on to do things like get a job or explore a hobby they would never have tried.

Despite being able to identify with the others who roomed in my house, there were still some people who made group home life difficult. In the house I first lived in back about 11 years before moving out, the first thing I encountered was a man around my age who was able to work and had a fancy new car that his dad had bought him, but was one of the most obnoxious people I have ever known. For some reason, I can't even begin to try and guess what his diagnosis was, but I had some information that he did too much LSD in his younger days, so perhaps that was why his brain and mouth had no filter between them. He would go up to people and ask them things like, "How's your piles?" Every once in a while, intrigued by the idea of driving his fancy new little sports car, I would volunteer to drive him to the bar where he could get drunk and not worry about an impaired charge. The only thing I had to worry about was being embarrassed to death by some of the things this guy would do. For example, he had a funny constitution and sometimes had trouble holding in his poop. The waitress would come and say, "Would you like a draft beer?"

His reply would come, plain as day, "Can't drink draft beer. Makes me shit my pants." One time I tried a Jedi mind trick on him and said,

"Oh come on. One won't hurt!" And his reply came, again very plainly,

"Yeah, maybe one won't hurt!" Then the next day invariably he tracked me down to say, "Thanks, Leif! I went and shit my pants again last night!" and I would nearly poop my own pants laughing at the absurdity-not only of him doing this but openly admitting to it.

That guy didn't last too long at our house. The staff moved him to the main house where the office and food were so they could supervise him better. There was still a guy who was a real problem. He was in his 50s or 60s and never changed his clothes or bathed. He would often do things like go out of his room to the bathroom with just a shirt on and no underwear and take a leak and then leave a trail of drips behind him. How he got so far down the food chain, I don't know because he was very handy at fixing all kinds of stuff and would help anyone. He had been an appliance repair person for years and had made decent money. His two kids seemed pretty much on the ball as well. I blame a poor diet for what happened to his health. He eventually died of colon cancer, and I was sad to see him go. I just didn't like living with someone who cared nothing for their hygiene or the cleanliness of a place I also have to live in.

I had quit smoking while I was still in the hospital but when I moved into the group home smoking was allowed inside our houses. In a short time, I was back on the cigarettes. I made the stupid mistake of keeping my last can of tobacco from when I smoked, and it was so easy just to sit down and start again. Now tobacco is priced very oppressively by the government. It costs about $10 for 20 cigarettes and even more to buy loose tobacco to roll your own. Smoking is a big thing for people with mental health issues. One of the people working at the group home was saying that a huge portion of cigarette sales are to people with mental health problems who only comprise a much smaller segment of the population than people without a mental illness. Just walking through the front doors of the building I was in at the psychiatric hospital, people would be out begging cigarettes, and the smoke in front of the doors was thick and stinking. There was an old lady there who would always say to people, "Do you have five dollars?" I don't know if she's still alive, but she's likely now asking for ten.

After the appliance guy and the `piles' guy had moved out, we got two new roommates. One was a man named Darren, and another was a younger person named Rich. Darren was my age, and I had attended school with him through the mental health clinic for a while, and we had been friends. Funny how friends at school don't always translate into good roommates. Darren ended up being a real jerk. Rich was a friend but very hard to deal with at times. He had a brain injury of some kind and would forget things from one minute to the next. Often I would be sitting rolling and smoking cigarettes and drinking coffee, and he would stand over me talking about the same things over and over. I'm surprised it didn't drive me to drink anything stronger.

Darren was another kettle of fish. I think he must have had schizophrenia, though I don't like to diagnose people. Darren was incredibly inconsiderate. He felt that if he wanted to play his music loud he had every right to do so. I tried to make it easier for him to listen to his music without bothering me. I even bought him a set of wireless headphones. One time before that he had been playing his music in his room so the whole house could hear and I went into the basement and cut off the power to his room and left it that way. He was mad as a hatter about it. Then we had a house meeting, and one of the staff was all upset that I had done this. So, trying to be a peacemaker, I got him the headphones and then one day he had them on, and he was singing on the main floor of the house at the top of his lungs. In his head, with the music directly next to his ears, it sounded good, but to everyone within earshot, it would have sounded better if someone tortured a cat in our living room. I yelled at him, but he kept singing. He even smiled at me as he was doing so. So I told him to shut the hell up, or I would cut the power again, and he righteously said, "You can't turn the power off. It's against the rules!" So of course, I shut the power down, and I don't think he did it again.

Rich was different. He was like a lost puppy dog to a lot of people, and I considered him a friend, but I strongly disagreed with a lot of things he did, like using and selling all the pot in the whole project. He often came to me and would bug me to borrow my video games, or my VCR, or money, or anything he could borrow. So I decided that I would lend things to him, but I had little respect for where his money originated. My solution to this moral dilemma was that I would charge him all I could reasonably charge, when anyone else would get these favors for free. After a while, it got to be that his monthly disability cheque would go to his room and board for the group home and then the rest would go to me. I hate to admit it, but he freely agreed to it and always paid me gladly knowing this way he didn't have to manage his money on his own. Time ticked away relatively fast from then on because I was always well fed and comfortable, and I had plenty of money to pursue my hobbies. Plus I even had a few friends. Maybe the best part of it, though, was that nearly every day my dad and I would go for long walks in the beautiful parks that line the river valley in Edmonton. There was something so therapeutic about doing that each day, and getting to know my dad like I did when I was younger.

Chapter Fifteen: Crying Sometimes Makes You Stronger

It is hard to believe how young I was when I think of my age now, and all the trouble I went through starting from my early teen years. My age didn't really seem to catch up to me until I hit 40. I've always been pretty athletic but as I have gotten older, I have been able to do less and less and needed more and more rest afterward. One of the things I got seriously into was swimming. I had always enjoyed it; the feeling of cool water rippling over you after spending long sweating minutes in a hot tub or sauna, the challenge of trying to push one more lap out of yourself as you fight to keep breathing enough to go on. Then there are all the little bonuses like socializing, sitting in the hot tub and all that. Not long after I settled into a routine at the group home, a year's pass for free to all city facilities was made available to me. It was hard at first to feel comfortable. I remember feeling embarrassed trying to talk with the other people who went to the same pool first thing in the morning. Then, after a while, I got to know the people who used the pool at the same time I did, and not only were all of them pretty friendly, but two of them were Danish and knew my dad's friends from St. Albert. They even gave me gifts on my birthday. It was great to get into shape, but also I was meeting new people and making new friends. It gave a lot of meaning to my days, and getting into shape allowed me to take on more jobs and balance my budget sooner than I thought I ever would.

I haven't yet talked much about interacting with my ex-girlfriend Debbie who I had met while attending school in Edmonton. The last time I got sick, and was put in hospital, she had decided that she couldn't have me in her life anymore. Every time I went by her old apartment building I thought about her and the times we had spent together. Sometimes we didn't get along, or there would be long periods of when we didn't talk, but then one day she would call me up for no reason, and we would talk long into the night. Sometimes she would also come over to my tiny apartment, and I would give her a massage, and we would spend more long hours together, and it was like we had never parted.

Then finally one day I built up the courage to go down and see her and she let me in, and we had a long talk. She was in tears because she had missed me too, but told me that it was just too hard for her to be friends with me as sick as I was. As a result of her saying I couldn't be trusted, I set out to prove to her that I could stay on my medications and treatment and be a good friend to her. I went to all of my doctor's visits. I took my medications, and especially, I was as honest as I could be about my mental health with my doctor and social worker. I put aside gambling and my other vices, even cigarettes. The staff at the mental health clinic were great people, though it wasn't them that had changed, it was my attitude towards them. As time passed, I even talked with them about Debbie and how I felt about her. After a while, still having a hard time getting down to see her and still having to wait for the odd chance that she would call me, I got her mailing address and decided to try to do what I do best: write. Every night I would sit down and write a long letter to her and include a poem in it that I had written right on the spot. Each time she would get one she would call me up, and I would go down and visit her again, so I kept on writing every day.

One night she called me up and was sorrowful. She had just gotten the news that her father had died. He had been something of an absent parent. Though he was in the room when she lived at his house, he showed no authority and said very little to anyone. Often he would drink up to 20 beers in a day and just sit quietly and smoke. Not long after I first met him he was taken to a treatment facility and then put into a psychiatric group home after a stay in the same hospital that had treated me. It was a sad way for a kind man and caring father to go. He had been a sheet metal worker for a long time and had provided a good income for his family. When Debbie was 14, and her parents had split up, she chose to drop out of school and live with her dad where there were no rules to speak of, and she could do pretty much what she wanted, which included drinking, and whatever else she felt like doing. I had met Debbie when she was trying to undo all those years of no discipline so she could finish school, and it ended up being too difficult for her. She dropped out twice before giving up.

When I would go over to visit Debbie after writing to her and waiting for her call, we would always go and buy the same order of wonton soup from a nearby Chinese place. It was fantastic food, and cheap. It became our routine soon enough, that we would eat this soup every night we got together. We must have had it 100 times at least. Not long after that Debbie got word that she was going to get an inheritance from her father, which was going to be at least $30,000. I felt happy for her and harbored a bit of joy, in that since I had shelled out so much money to keep her going over the years, there was now a possibility of the favors being reciprocated. Sadly, when she got the money she cut off all contact with me again. I spent the next few months missing her, time which I filled up reading Steinbeck and eating too much. When she finally got back in touch with me I learned that the $30,000 had been spent- mostly on crack. I was appalled. If I had heard she had done that from anyone but herself, I would not have believed it. But apparently, she had a job in a bakery with a really evil guy who used to keep her working 30 or 40 hours at a time and would feed her the drugs to keep her going.

My life had been developing a bit during Debbie's absence as well, though. I had gotten a job as a security guard and had soon saved up enough money to travel to Toronto to visit my sister for the first time. The last time I had seen her was when I was in the hospital in 2001 and was very sick. Little did I know that she and my Dad had been fighting all kinds of bureaucracy to try and get me better treatment, and to get me out of that horrible lockdown ward in the mental hospital. Visiting her was the high point of that part of my life. Toronto was sunny and beautiful, my sister and I got along great. There were so many new things to see and do there. After a few days, she introduced me to her boyfriend and his two daughters. Her boyfriend was a recovering alcoholic/drug addict and had grown up wealthy and privileged. These things made for a pretty abrasive combination in a person, but once I learned he was intelligent and easy going, and an incredible cook, I decided he was better than the abusive Greek communist she used to have as a boyfriend.

One of the cooler things we did was to go to the top of the CN Tower in Toronto, and I think at the time it was the second tallest human-made structure in the world. The view was incredible. Toronto is perhaps the biggest city I have ever been to, except London. I think it tops five million people and the downtown skyline blows away anything I've seen, including Los Angeles. Part of the observation deck on the famous tower has a glass floor, and though they say it could hold the weight of a rhinoceros, few people dared step onto it knowing they could look straight down about 4,000 feet to the ground below. I walked on it but not for very long.

My sister and I took a lot of walks and bus rides, and even some ferry rides to islands out in Lake Ontario. I have always loved being on boats out over the water; somehow it symbolized freedom to me. The best boat ride we took of the trip was when we went to see Niagara Falls, and we took a little ferry boat called "The Maid of the Mist" right up to the edge of the falls.

When we got back, my sister had made a comment that she thought it was strange that I called our dad every day, but to me, it wasn't. That hospital stay had taken all the courage and self-will right out of me. Day after day, month after month of incarceration and beatings, and being locked in the isolation room made me into a little kid again inside. I needed my dad, and anyone I could get for support, to talk to every day. I still don't know what I will do when my dad gets too old to go out and do things with me or passes away. My sister and I have something of an unwritten agreement that when that happens, I will move to Toronto, but I don't know if that will be possible.

I went home to my security guard job in which I worked at a palliative care hospital. I had become friends with three nurses, one of which had a boyfriend in the army and nearly talked me into trying to join up. The two other nurses that I met were best friends. One of them was single and a bit of a princess, and the other was married with three kids-her name was Ruby. I have to confess that I developed something of a schoolboy crush on Ruby, the married woman with three kids. I think she liked me too, but it would be a terrible thing to let an infatuation break up a marriage and put kids through the whole concept of having a temporary father figure and all that, so I never even implied to her how I felt about her.

Working there, as in other places before, I had people confront me and tell me how to do my job. One of these people complained right to my boss that I didn't ask him for ID when he came in, despite the fact that the hospital was a public place where anyone is free to go unless they have been banned. Then there was another guy who felt that I was slack in my duties by drinking coffee while working. I have always known that a cup of coffee in your hand can save your life in security work. It helps keep you alert, and can be used in a defensive capacity though I have never had to do so. But these people kept complaining about me, and how I should do my job, so I simply quit just like I had done with so many other jobs. End of problem.

A few months later, I got word that my disability pension, The Assured Income For The Severely Handicapped, or AISH, which had been taking money off my monthly disbursements for years was ruled to have done so illegally. So, after a lot of waiting, I was sent a cheque totaling $8,000, and I was in heaven for a little while. I bought a car first off, and by now Debbie had made the decision (thank god!) to get away from the drugs and her boss, and moved up to a small town way north of Edmonton with her mom. For a while, I was driving up all that way whenever I could, to visit and encourage her. Like anything good in my life it didn't last.

By chance, a job application that I had put in for a well-paying job came through, so all of a sudden-for the first time in my life-I had a little money. The job was originally for work as a security guard on movie sets, but after a few days of working in a non-heated hospital in winter, I decided I couldn't handle it. By some luck, they had another job available setting up concerts. When I asked what their wage was, I nearly dropped the phone because they paid twice the money I had ever gotten.

I tried out the concert job. My first concert was a band called Tool, and I was just about ready to give up after one shift. The physical labor nearly killed me. After considering the money, though, and that it wasn't a full-time job, I decided to work out on my off days so I could stick with it. So I soon moved out of the group home, mostly because they told me since they were subsidized housing and that subsidized housing charges 30% of your income, they would have to raise my rent to something like $1,000 a month which was preposterous.

I moved into an unsupervised house for people with mental health issues for a flat rate, and as summer rolled around I bought a motorcycle and, after getting in an accident in my car, I bought a flashy red Honda Sports car.

The new home I moved to seemed pretty good at first. I knew one of the guys from being in the hospital with him, and I knew he was a blowhard. He was always trying to push people around, prove how tough he was. So I was able to stay on his good side by avoiding any implications that he wasn't the toughest guy in the world, or the smartest and so on. There was another guy there who was perhaps the one person I have ever met who likely should have been permanently kept in an institution for life. His name was Lewis, and there was something very seriously wrong with him. I think he would have scored high on a sociopath test, but I didn't know it at first. I tried to take him under my wing. I hung out with him for a while (he had been my brother's roommate for a while) and then stopped, then ran into him again at an 'Anonymous' meeting and so I thought he was not only reaching out for help but had the ability to improve his life. Once again, I couldn't have been more wrong about someone. I remember giving him ride after ride, taking him to visit his mom, and his mom trying to warn me that he was beyond help. One of the red flags came up when he said that he was paying back his Dad because he had smashed up his car. Everyone who didn't hear the whole story assumed he meant he had borrowed the car and got in an accident. No, this guy had taken an ax and went about completely destroying a brand new car with it. He also told me that at one point he had been in the same ward in the hospital I was in and went out and got as drunk as possible. When he came back, a nurse came up to talk to him, and he backhanded her and said, 'I hate everything to do with psychiatry!' and was put into the forensics ward the very next day. I have to say that Lewis' problem is very rare, and his main issue likely had more to do with alcohol and drug abuse than his diagnosis of a mental illness.

I lived at that place for quite a while regardless of all the problems, but finally, Adam, the same person I had known years before in the University Hospital who thought he was Superman drove me out. I was in the kitchen, and he was standing over the stove, and I reached above his head to open a cupboard but stopped, waiting for him to move so I could open it. He wouldn't move, though, so I just opened it. He looked at me with anger and yelled, "Say excuse me!" and I only said "No." Then he started to fly into a rage and was yelling and threatening me. He said I was acting like a baby. I told him he was the one acting like a baby and he said, "If you want proof of my manhood I invite you to step outside!" In no way was I going to do this. He had a way of doing these things: no matter what the outcome he would benefit. If you backed down, he would make sure and ride you harder the next time. If you agreed to fight and beat the crap out of him, he would charge you with assault.

So despite the fact that he got the woman from downstairs to beg me not to call the police, I did anyways just to make sure, and somehow he sweet-talked the cops into thinking it was just a little mistake on my part. The next day I phoned up the landlord to get him kicked out and he refused. He wanted to move me to the house he owned that my brother lived in, but I knew the place was a drug den with a practicing prostitute in it. I went to my nurse, and she found a much better place back in my old part of town, and I put my present landlord down as a reference. When he got word that I was moving, he went even more ballistic than the guy who lived in the basement. He came down, used his key to open my door and came in kicking things around and yelling at me. That made it inevitable I was going to move out. I ended up with a fairly nice apartment but little did I know the place was full of people even more unstable than those in the group home.

Chapter Sixteen: No Place To Call Home

I moved into my new small apartment and felt a certain sense of security that this was a regular place, governed by law, and that it was my own. The only problem was that I shared a bathroom with one other person, and I think he might have been a meth head, though I know little about the subject. He would hear me at any hour opening the door to the bathroom and he would open the door and talk and talk until I just wanted him to shut up so I could go. He kept trying to tell me there was a gas leak in the building and that he was going to sue for some untold amount of money. I honestly hope he wasn't smoking meth in there because the fumes would have gone through the door and started to affect me.

At the time I had made friends with a young woman from work who was from Australia and, little did I know, I was way too much for her. I would write her long emails and give her books I thought she would like and stuff. I think the big thing I did wrong was to try to make her out to be the friend Debbie was, when in reality she wasn't emotionally available for that kind of friendship with someone. The crux of things came when she took a trip to Australia and didn't call for a month. I went through so much pain and regret during that time. When I did get to the point of prying the truth out of her, she admitted that things had gone too far and she didn't know how I would react if she were honest with me. That ended up making me feel horrible. I think that was the last time I actively sought after a life partner. From then on I stopped going to bars and other places and stopped trying at all to look for 'Mrs. Right.' The funniest thing was that not long after that I got to be close with a young woman, and this friendship had nearly as much genuine feeling that I had with Debbie.

She was a young woman from my home town who worked as a chef. Like Debbie, she had her issues, but I didn't want to judge her because of that. She had a hard-edged side to her, but growing up in St. Albert like we did, I understood that completely. Not to say she was a princess; she was an unyielding young woman with high standards, and I think, sadly, I didn't meet all of them. We used to hang out quite a bit. She was an English Major in University, and I was a writer. I felt it made for a good fit, but we were just friends for the whole time that we knew each other. She was sincere and intelligent and had these pretty dark eyes that a person could just lose themselves in. If she were late for work, I would pick her up with an energy drink ready for her. If she needed a ride at 3 am, I would go without hesitation. In the middle of our friendship she was living with her boyfriend, and for some reason, he kept fighting with her while she was trying to study, she just had one more exam to graduate, and her degree had taken her six years to accomplish. She called me, but I didn't have a car at the time, so I called her a cab, paid for it when it got to my house, and set up my computer for her to study. A few days later she found out that she had passed by the skin of her teeth. She was going to have me escort her to her graduation but, after a while, she decided to take her dad instead. That wasn't all that bad, but over the time we were friends it seemed she made a lot of promises that she never kept.

Going to the clinic I started hearing some interesting things about what my psychopath friend (Lewis from the house I lived in previously) was doing. Apparently one day he got drunk out of his mind, walked into the living room and took a whiz right up against the wall. He kept calling me for rides, too. I would try and say no, but then he would say things like, "But you're my only normal friend!" or "I feel better after I talk to you." I have to admit that when I was living in that small bachelor apartment with my only social outlet either work or going to the pool, I broke down and went to visit him or do things with him. I had been a bit freaked out because near the end of my term as his roommate he had tried to kill himself. Another time he hitch-hiked to Jasper, the mountain resort town, and tried to find a job dishwashing while he was missing one shoe. Social Services somehow convinced him to head back to Edmonton and put him on a Greyhound. How this guy managed to stay out of the grave defies me. I often wonder where he is now.

Living in a small bachelor suite by myself again slowly started to wear me down. I did have one more social outlet: my dad and brother. I lavished them with gifts and meals out, and all kinds of things. At one point my brother came up to me at the flea market and told me he had just seen an incredible guitar on sale for only $300 and seemed surprised when I handed him the cash. On a different occasion I bought my dad a gold watch and a fancy camera. Then my sister came to visit one time, and while everyone looked at me she told me the news-I was going to be an uncle. I couldn't ever have been happier. A few months later she gave birth to a beautiful, happy little girl she named Willomena who has been the light of my life ever since. I have a picture I cherish of her: 3 years old and sitting on the back of my motorbike, happy and smiling with her beautiful curly-head mop shining in the sun. Her incredible imagination inspired me to write a children's chapter book about her and some fictional people from other planets. She had been born with a cleft palette and I worked that into the book as a lesson for kids to accept others who have differences.

Downstairs from me, there was a guy who claimed to have a lot of construction knowledge who went on and on about how much money he was going to make after going to our local technical institute. He even got his picture put on a billboard advertising the college, but he didn't last long there. They told him they didn't want to see him come back until he had consulted a psychiatrist, and it was easy enough to understand why. He used to go on about how he had all these biker friends who wanted to induct him into some big outlaw biker gang. Some of his stories were entertaining and could have been true, but the problem with him came in another form. For some reason, the house was sold, and the new owner gave him a job renovating one of his other buildings, collecting the rent, and vacuuming the carpets in the place where I lived. There were only six suites, and he didn't even get his suite for free in the agreement, but, soon after, he went around giving orders and serving notices like he owned the place. One day I came home, and he was just leaving my suite and locking the door-for no stated purpose. I moved out, and then six months later my mail-forwarding agreement with the post office ended. I had forgotten to update one address, and despite that I phoned him and went down to pick it up, he sent my cheque back to Canada Pension Plan's office as though I had committed some fraud.

On the advice of my sister, I moved back to the multi-house group home which made a world of difference. There are more rules to follow, but I think having friends, lowered stress about having enough food, and paying all the bills helped me a great deal.

For some years my mom had been in bad health. When I was around 20, it was hard to accept but a serious problem with her back forced her to be confined to a wheelchair. She had needed an operation for a crushed vertebra in her neck in which they took bone from her hip to make a space around the crushed bone in the back of her neck, having to go past her esophagus and carotid arteries. It was touch and go for a while, but she got through it.

Years went by and her back one day started giving her so much pain she could hardly leave her bed. Her quality of life grew worse and worse, and for a long time, she needed to be on oxygen because of a problem with her lungs. There were times when she seemed to do better, but as the years went on her psychiatric health also grew worse. This degeneration of someone I loved was very hard for me to take. I wanted somehow to help anyone I could who had problems like mine, and here was my mom getting worse, with nothing for me to do at all but give her small comforts. I would visit often, call often, and once I talked my dad into putting a TV in their bedroom so she could have something to keep her mind off things.

A number of years after I got out of the hospital myself, and also after my niece had been born, my Dad was invited to attend my sister's wedding to her long-time boyfriend and father of her child, Willa. There was no question of me being the one to stay behind and take care of my Mom when he was away. There was no one else except maybe my brother, but he didn't have a driver's license. The job was not an easy one. I had done it before, providing 24-hour care to someone with poor health. I had to give meals, snacks, adjust her in bed, give medications and apply creams, and help her to the bathroom. Despite all of my help, twice she went into such a panic that she had me call an ambulance, and the paramedics chastised me for keeping my Mom in a self-contained apartment. It was my dad's call on that one, but we all knew if we put her in a home she wouldn't get the care needed and she would be miserable. Then the worst happened.

I was sitting in the living room of my parents' apartment, and all I heard was my mom's cry, the last thing she would ever say: the child's version of my name, "Leify." I went into her room, and she was waving her hands, and I looked at her confused, wondering what she was about to say, what she was trying to tell me. I put my hand on her chest and suddenly realized I had better call 911, which I did. I was in a bit of a panic. They asked me first if she was breathing and after checking, I realized she wasn't. Right over the phone they gave me quick instructions in CPR - something I had trained in years ago but had forgotten how to administer. I dragged her onto the floor, and just got in a couple of breaths before the paramedics got there. They dragged her into the foyer of the small apartment and went to work. A black cloud descended over me. I knew that even if they got her going there would be serious problems with her back after being man-handled and chest-compressed. After trying for a few minutes, the head paramedic at the scene - there was at least four of them - told me I should use this last chance to lean down and say my last words to her. I whispered a few words of love and inspiration as best I could and went back to the living room while I heard them try to resuscitate her.

A few minutes later they got my mom on a gurney and the head paramedic drove me to the hospital in a separate truck. He hemmed and hawed a bit but basically told me that my mom was 'no more' as the natives say. I got to the hospital and the staff got me a private room with a phone and some tissue, and I talked with the doctors and agreed there was no point in keeping her alive. She had been through so much in her life, from her early days as an impoverished and abused child, to months spent in psychiatric wards and hospitals from the age of 16 on, to untold amounts of pain from her back and other complaints that were so severe a doctor had consented to allow her opium suppositories, the last hope of those with no hope. Now it was time for her to rest.

They let me sit next to her as they shut down the respirator and she kept breathing for a short period. She looked so alive; her eyes were wide open. I tried to close them but they kept opening and I almost wanted to tell someone she was still kicking, but I knew in my heart it didn't mean that at all. I held her hand and in a few minutes it was done. I phoned my dad and my brother and all I could think about was my sister from now on thinking of her wedding day as the day her mom died. I also felt incredible guilt that of all the times she could have gone she went while I was supposed to be taking care of her. I was destroyed.

I think in a lot of ways I have fulfilled what my mom would have wanted for me. She knew I had a mental illness, which caused a very special bond between us. What she didn't know at the time was that if I took my medications, if I worked hard, I could do as well as anyone. In the past few years I have written and published more than ten books, and books were something precious to my mom, she loved her literature. It hurts when I look back and think of some of the things I did that only caused my mom more pain and worry, like taking off hitch-hiking, going to flight school while I was off medication, and trying to join the military during the Gulf War. Somehow I have been able to grow past all of that, and now my family is the most important thing in my life. My mom would be proud of the legacy she left the world. A daughter who succeeded at my mom's biggest dream of becoming a teacher, as well as a granddaughter who is so happy and giving and intelligent. A son (my brother) who has shown incredible strength, courage, and talent as he faces a serious health issue and continues to live his life. I like to think I can be added to this list as well, having built a small amount of fame as a writer and a good reputation as a public speaker concerning mental health issues, and a teacher of creative writing and wellness recovery classes.

When I was young, my sister was the light of my life, and now as I approach middle age, her daughter has filled that role. There were some tough times between my sister and I. For an extended period she saw me as just more trouble in her life that she didn't need. We have since become much closer, as the short years that separate our ages mean less and family bonds mean more. I have been out to Toronto now five or six times and I am happy to say I could never have been more proud of the life my sister has made for herself through hard work and intelligence.

My hope for the future is that I will be able to continue sharing the message that mental illness is not something to be afraid of, or to be hushed into dark corners. Stigma has a real and severe effect on both people who live with a mental illness, and those have a loved one or friend who is affected. This makes me feel I have to keep writing; I have to keep giving talks. I have spoken now to dozens of gatherings and classes that I hope will make a difference, from police recruit classes to university psychiatric nursing classes, all the way down through high school and junior high. The greatest reward I have known from doing this was when I spoke to a high school class, and a young woman who had no idea anything was wrong but had been feeling troubled, came forward to talk to the other presenter and me after class. She was able to connect with resources, and I hope and pray that she was able to find help. I often wonder about all of the wreckage and torment I left behind when I was sick, willfully off medications. Experiences like I had with that girl who came forward helps me to feel more whole, more justified in my existence. I have a lot of things in my life I want to make up for.

There are so many things a person needs to understand about their illness to manage it properly. The first thing of course is to communicate. If you see the warning signs of mental illness in yourself or a loved one, talk about your feelings and thoughts with a doctor or someone you trust. Reach out and find the help you need. Thanks to advances in knowledge and technology and medications, many people these days don't even have to ever see the inside of a psychiatric facility, they are treated and managed in their own community. A psychiatrist is your best first step if possible. Then take your medications just as prescribed, at the same time each day. Give it time to work and don't go off any of it without talking to your doctor first. Then find a place where you can be accepted and understood as a person who needs treatment. Build a community, online and offline, of people you can talk with, though you may want to share your mental health issues only with a professional. Above all, believe that mental health and wellness can be a reality. I may have gone through a lot, had a lot of good and bad in my life, but now mental health is my priority, and it makes a huge difference.

A few days after my mom passed, we had a quiet service in the mountains that she loved to be around with no priest or pastor, we just scattered her ashes that were mixed with the ashes of her favorite Teddy Bear, Fred, and we each said what words we could. I often think as I look back on becoming an adult, the transition seems to have more to do with understanding that we don't live as an island, really. We depend so much upon each other, and when we lose someone close to us, especially when it's beyond our control, we either grow or let the loss destroy us. My loss nearly wrecked me but now I go on, thinking of what losing me, or her mother, would mean to my niece and how important it is to soldier on-no matter what.

Mother's Day Without Our Mom

Mother's Day is the time
When something special must come to be
A well-cooked meal, a little wine
To make that special Mother see

See that as the years went past
We only need them more and more
And though they may no longer be in charge
We love them like before

I watched my little niece one time
Look at my sister with a glowing smile
And thought how sad it is that kind of love
Seems to only last a while

When I had my Mom here on Earth
She loved me true and never let me down
She was there to call when I needed strength
And no others were around

When I was a young young boy
Coming home from a schoolyard fight
She let me know that at least one person cared
Though my loss was all the school's delight

And now I draw upon her strength
Though she has moved on up above

Let us all try and fill our hearts and minds
With our wonderful mothers' love

Leif Gregersen, May 11, 2013

Afterword to the second edition, February 1, 2017:

Losing my mom was hard on every member of my family. When we were arranging her affairs, I got a chance to look at her high school yearbook and she looked so young and happy in her picture. Someone had written about her that "Bev studies so hard she won't be happy until she's a teacher herself." My mom would have become a teacher but just as I would have become a soldier or a pilot or a lawyer, mental illness got in the way. This was something I felt I shared with my mom that no one else did but my sister, my brother and my dad each had special things they shared with my mom.

I often wonder when my real recovery from mental illness began. Was it at the end of my six-month stay in the hospital? Did it begin when I came back from Vancouver? I read recently that recovery is a process and it doesn't always happen in a linear fashion. You can make progress and then go back in the hospital and start over, but you don't always start over from scratch. Many things happened that helped me along the way. Perhaps the most important was going into a supportive group home. The staff there were incredible, they had such compassion and caring and helped me in every way. There were times when I did nothing but read Steinbeck and eat, and no one put any pressure or expectations on me. I just had to take my medications, see my doctor and stay well. I think without this situation existing for me I wouldn't have recovered nearly to the point of functioning as I do now.

I also have my dad to thank. He has been such a kind person to me and now that I am older I realize that he had done so much for me way before I ever got sick. As a young child I loved him so dearly and now that my sister has a daughter I am amazed at how his caring and compassion and sense of fun and joy has remained. In a way I always wanted to become a writer for my dad, him and my mom put so much emphasis on good literature. I recall a time when I was around 10 and loved reading comic books of all kinds and he had me read of all things, a short novel by John Steinbeck. I think now that I have published books and know popular authors as friends that he is very proud of me. I worry about every little thing that happens to him, I know he won't be around forever, I just pray that when he does go I will be strong enough and have enough support to keep going without him.

When I first wrote this book I had a lot of anger in me, but things have changed. It does no good for someone to blame others for your relationship status, your finances, your living standards. A person has to one day take stock of what they have been doing in relationships, employment, self-care and sweep their own side of the walk. For a long time I blamed others for all of these things and more. The fact is that I am incredibly blessed with good friends and a wonderful family and community. Over time I have been able to develop myself in many ways from working a steady job to becoming a better photographer which has helped me to earn enough money to buy not just what I need, but also things I want. I never thought it was possible, but in 2016 I accomplished something so incredible my heart still leaps with joy each time I think of it. I made it to London, England. I only went for 9 days, but I basked in all the sights and sounds of when my dad took my brother and I there as kids and I got to experience history from right up close.

I make mention of two young women in particular that I seemed to be 'stuck' on. I like to try and emphasize that I never had any kind of relationship with them, but my delusions made me think they were controlling my thoughts and were toying with me. In reality they are just two ordinary people who want to be left alone. I hate to say it, but in this case, my medications don't do the full job I wish they could. I still have invasive thoughts about these women, and other things that are based on a milder form of psychosis that my medication just doesn't deal with. I may never have perfect mental health, but over the years I have learned to be able to focus my scattered thoughts and concentrate like a person without a mental illness. A few years back I wanted to try and talk to these two women just so I could go to my high school reunion, but I was given a plain 'no' in response. The truth is I feel awful about the whole thing and I actually have a lot of gratitude for them for not having me charged with harrasment or something else sinister like having someone assault me. The best thing I can do is to try to think about other things when thoughts of them or strange ideas pop into my head.

As far as relationships go, I still talk with Debbie each and every day though she lives out of town. We have a strong connection to each other based on real caring and it is a very special thing to me. I have come to accept not having a romantic relationship and just working on my writing and my recovery at this point. I also have a few more close friends from high school days who have helped immensely with my writing and my self-esteem.

One of the more important things that happened in my recovery was that I made more of an effort to look into Buddhism and how it could help train me to control my thoughts. For a while I was reading all I could and even went to a Tibetan Monk living in Edmonton to learn to meditate. It helped me find new limits to stress levels and also helped me to calm some of the anger I have in me that comes out in rude remarks and frustration with other people at times. The process is so simple, but there is enough information involved to spend a lifetime studying the subject. It all comes down to the essential function of breathing. Breathing is the most spiritual thing one can do, taking in lungfuls of air and processing it to feed your mind and body. You turn off all your personal monitoring systems, you clear your thoughts and just let yourself be guided by a gentle control of your breath. Once you practise this for a while, you become more focused, you can better control your emotions, and happiness isn't so difficult to conceive of.

It is hard to say what my initial intentions were in writing "Through the Withering Storm" and this book. I liked the idea of making money from telling my story, I wanted to record my life. It has become so much more than that. Over the past two years, I have been taking classes and giving presentations about the journey from illness through recovery to mental health as a lived experience presenter for the Schhizophrenia Society. Just yesterday I taught a group of 12 adults who have the illness the first of a series of five classes regarding recovery and wellness. I felt such compassion for the men and women there, I felt a true connection that they were at different stages of life that I had been in. I was so amazed to find out that many of the people there had done just as much as I had in their lives but needed to find a way to manage their illness. It feels odd to say, but in just one class I felt a strong bond with these people.

The other job I do for the Schizophrenia Society is giving talks about mental illness and my own personal story for university classes, police recruit classes, high school and junior high classes. In all honesty I never thought I would get up in front of a lecture hall full of people and talk comfortably about things that went wrong with my mind and the importance of everyone understanding mental illness. As a youth of fourteen, I was a patient on a psychiatric ward and while I was there I was allowed to go to Air Cadets where I had to give a speech in front of just a few of my peers and I had an almost psychotic nervousness. I could barely speak, I was shaking, I had a hard time holding my head up. The thing that makes me feel so good is that now not only am I able to get up in front of many people and share my life experience in hopes of helping others understand mental illness, but in a way I am doing something that my mom would have been very proud of, I am a teacher.

Another thing that makes me feel a great sense of joy is that my sister has given my family the incredible joy of a child we all love dearly. Not only that, but as time has passed and I have worked hard at my recovery, taking medications regularly, keeping informed about my condition and staying on top of things, my sister has fully let me back into her life. She now has a house in

Toronto and I have gone to visit her and my niece on several occasions.

I think a large part of how far I have come has to do with a union that I worked for over the past ten years. It is the union that handles labor for entertainment, and I loved just about every minute of the time I spent with them. Before the last time I was ill and went to the hospital, I had a hard time keeping a job for a few months. Now I have held a job for ten years and made many lasting friendships and enough money to travel and finance the publication of my books. I no longer work for the union, but I am still in good standing on their books and can go back any time I want. Working in entertainment, as a security guard on movie sets, as a stage hand, truck loader and many other tasks has done a great deal of good for my self-esteem.

A few short months ago I was called in to the office of the group home I had been living in. The lady in charge, who had been more a friend than just a project manager, but a friend, told me that the group home was no longer supporting me. She made arrangements for me to get my own apartment in a building close by. I liked that I would be staying in the community, but I wasn't sure about living alone. For all the rules and frustrations that the group home had that I didn't get along with, there was a sense of community there. I moved into my own place in September of 2016 and now it is January and I am very happy. I have my own kitchen and fridge and my own space to do what I like in. I have my dad, my cousin, and some friends over often. There is even an office where we can go and drink coffee and interact with other residents and staff if they are not too busy.

Life has become so much more for me than the life I had 15 years ago when I left the psychiatric hospital. Every day I have to remind myself to stay grounded though. I need my medications, I need the injection that keeps my thoughts clear every two weeks. I need to feed my body, feed my mind and exercise. I also need to care for and give respect to each individual I encounter. My illness is now just a small part of my life, but it can grow and fester at any time. I also have to be grounded and be aware that it has now been over five years since I had a drink of any kind, it has been three since I gambled, and thirteen years since I smoked tobacco or anything else. Like my friend used to say, we haven't got a cure, we have a daily reprieve from our affliction based on the maintenance of our spiritual condition

Made in the USA
Columbia, SC
01 November 2020